OFFICE OF POPULATION CENSUSES AN...

FOR REFERENCE USE ONLY

Series MB1 no. 19

Cancer statistics
registrations

Cases of diagnosed cancer registered in England and Wales, 1986

Microfiche

London: HMSO

© *Crown Copyright 1991*
Applications for reproduction should be made to HMSO
First published 1991

ISBN 0 11 691349 5

Contents

	Page
List of tables	iv
Introduction	1
Scope, method and use of the cancer registration scheme	1
Trends in cancer incidence	2
Cancer registrations	3
Annual registration tables	3
Survival tables	3
Validity of statistics	3
The ten most common cancer sites	3
Cumulative risk of cancer registration	4
Definitions	5
Cancer	5
Populations	5
Regional health authorities	5
Predominantly urban and predominantly rural aggregations	7
Standardised registration ratio	8
Symbols and conventions used	8
Further information	8
Acknowledgement	8
References	8
Envelope containing microfiche	Inside back cover

List of tables

			Page
Table 1	Standardised registration ratios (base year 1979): sex and site 1977-1986*	England and Wales	9
Table 2	Registrations of newly diagnosed cases of cancer: sex, site and age, 1986	England and Wales	14
Table 3	Rates per 100,000 population of newly diagnosed cases of cancer: sex, site and age, 1986	England and Wales	22
Table 4	Registrations of newly diagnosed cases of cancer: sex, site (4 digit breakdown of ICD 9th Revision) and age, 1986	England and Wales	fiche
Table 5	Rates per 100,000 population of newly diagnosed cases of cancer: sex, site (4 digit breakdown of ICD 9th Revision) and age, 1986	England and Wales	fiche
Table 6	All age crude rate and directly age standardised rates per 100,000 population of newly diagnosed cases of cancer: sex and site (4 digit breakdown of ICD 9th Revision), 1986	England and Wales	30
Table 7	Registrations of newly diagnosed cases of cancer: sex and site, 1986	England and Wales, regional health authorities	48
Table 8	Standardised registration ratios : sex and site, 1986	England and Wales, regional health authorities	56
Table 9	Directly age standardised (world standard population) rates of newly diagnosed cases of cancer: sex and site, 1986	England and Wales, regional health authorities	64
Table 10	Registrations of newly diagnosed cases of cancer: sex and site, 1986	England and Wales, standard regions, metropolitan counties, predominantly urban aggregates and predominantly rural aggregates	fiche
Table 11	Standardised registration ratios: sex and site, 1986	England and Wales, standard regions, metropolitan counties, predominantly urban aggregates and predominantly rural aggregates	fiche
Table 12	Directly age standardised (world standard population) rates for newly diagnosed cases of cancer: sex and site, 1986	England and Wales, standard regions, metropolitan counties, predominantly urban aggregates and predominantly rural aggregates	fiche

* 1977, 1978 and 1980-84 figures relate to persons aged under 75. Figures for 1985 and 1986 relate to persons of all ages.

			Page
Appendix A	Estimated resident population: sex and age, as at 30 June 1986	England and Wales, England, Wales, regional health authorities, metropolitan counties, predominantly urban aggregates and predominantly rural aggregates	72
Appendix B	Registrations of newly diagnosed cases of cancer: area of registration and area of residence, 1986	England and Wales, regional health authorities	76
Appendix C	Cancer incidence to mortality ratios: sex and site, 1986	England and Wales, regional health authorities	78

Introduction

Cancer statistics 1986 presents data, for England and Wales, on those patients who were first diagnosed with cancer in 1986 and who were registered by 31 May 1991. Comparable statistics for England and Wales for 1971 to 1985 have been published in the *Cancer statistics* (Series MB1) reports. For data prior to 1971, statistics have been published in the *Registrar General's Statistical Review of England and Wales, Supplements on Cancer*.

In England and Wales there has been a scheme for the registration of cancer patients since 1945. This scheme is voluntary and closely follows recommendations made by the 1980 Advisory Committee on Cancer Registration[1] in agreement with regional cancer registries. In 1989, the Registrar General's Medical Advisory Committee appointed a working party to review again cancer registration in England and Wales. The report of this review[2] contains detailed descriptions of the regional and national cancer registration schemes.

Scope, method and use of the cancer registration scheme

Cancer registration is the process of maintaining a systematic collection of data on the occurrence and characteristics of malignant neoplasms (and certain other neoplasms which are either pre-malignant or neoplasms of sites where distinguishing malignant from other neoplasms is difficult).

All patients diagnosed as suffering from cancer in England and Wales have been, or should have been, registered by cancer registries. Patients who were registered abroad, have no fixed abode, or whose address is either not stated or, if stated the location is not known, are excluded from all tables apart from Appendix B. In general, each of the cancer registries covers the area controlled by the regional health authorities (RHAs) in England and the registries record details for patients living within their respective areas. The Welsh Office is responsible for the registration of patients resident in Wales. Cancer registries are notified by the Office of Population Censuses and Surveys (OPCS) of any deaths in their area where cancer is mentioned on the death certificate. This facility is used to identify patients not previously known to the registries.

The national cancer registration scheme provides for the cancer registries to submit notifications of registered patients to OPCS by means of magnetic tape. These are computer processed, edited and the data are then transferred to annual OPCS magnetic tape files on which the following statistical information is held:

Registration identifying particulars
Usual residence area code
Birthplace code
Date of birth and age at registration
Sex
Occupation, status and industry codes (patient)
Occupation, status and industry codes (husband/father)
Primary tumour site code
Histological type and behaviour codes
Anniversary date
Date of death or date last known alive
Duration of survival
Expanded area code of usual residence
Postcode
Multiple tumour indicator
Death registration particulars (ie. registration district, sub-district and entry number)
Social class
Socio-economic group

Since 1971, cancer registrations have been recorded in the National Health Service Central Register (NHSCR), Southport. Deaths of all persons are routinely recorded in this register and a special note is made when the death of a cancer patient occurs. In this way, routine mortality follow-up information is provided by the NHSCR. OPCS magnetic tapes are updated with this death information in order to produce statistical analyses of cancer survival. Details of any death from causes other than cancer for registered patients known to NHSCR are also regularly sent to each regional cancer registry.

At its simplest, the aim of the scheme is to achieve a central register of all patients who develop malignancy. The uses to which such a system can be put may be summarised as:

Epidemiological studies, which may be descriptive or hypothesis testing;
management planning of services for cancer prevention and for cancer patients;
medical care studies;
studies of survival from malignant disease.

Quite different from the applications of the published statistics, there is continuing opportunity for individuals (research workers and others) to request ad hoc analyses from the national files - which again may be for descriptive or analytic purposes. A very different category of work is the use of the information about individuals developing malignant disease, to serve either as a point for retrospective studies or as an end point in historical prospective studies (particularly by way of the facility offered to follow-up individuals through the NHSCR). Further discussion of the uses of cancer registration are beyond the scope of this limited comment.

Trends in cancer incidence

The standardised registration ratios (see definition on page 8) by sex and site for the calendar period 1977-86 are presented in **Table 1**. The SRRs have been calculated using 1979 as the base year for the standardisation and are based on the Ninth Revision of the ICD.[3] Caution must be expressed about the difficulty of interpreting time trends of cancer registrations. The comments about validity below indicate that these statistics cannot immediately be interpreted as statistics of cancer incidence in the community. Variation in the completeness of diagnosis or the reporting of diagnosed cases to regional registries can alter the statistics, independently of any genuine change in the incidence of the malignancy. Also, longer time trends are required to probe specifically the major trends that exist in the different malignancies.

The use of SRRs has the advantage that the data for a particular site and sex can be presented as one index figure, rather than the need to examine age-specific rates for 5- or 10- year age-groups. However, if the age-specific trends in registration rates are different at different age-groups, the use of an SRR will be a distorting factor. A major addition to the material available for examination of trends in incidence is the publication on cancer surveillance[4], which can be purchased direct from OPCS from the address on page 8. This publication presents data for the span 1968-78, and gives the age-specific numbers and rates of registration for both sexes, site by site, together with a test of significance of the trend based on the years 1975-78. The test of significance is limited to the later part of the time span. There was appreciable alteration in registration in 1974-75, when registration of patients dying with malignant disease for whom no further information was available began.

Bearing the above comments in mind, the following points can be made in relation to **Table 1**. For all malignant neoplasms there are no marked trends over the period. When specific sites of malignancy are examined there are some trends of note (in addition there are some sites for which it is difficult to distinguish trend from chance fluctuations due to small numbers of registrations).

Lung cancer registrations (when adjusted for age) have decreased for males but increased for females over the period 1977-86. Malignant melanoma of the skin SRRs for 1986 show increases on those for 1985, for both sexes, and there has been an overall increase during 1977-86. Stomach cancer SRRs have decreased over the period 1977-86. There have been marked downward secular trends in SRRs for cancers coded to lymphosarcoma and reticulosarcoma and to Hodgkin's disease but a contrary trend for those coded to other malignant neoplasm of lymphoid and histiocytic tissue to which less well specified lymphomas would be coded. Testis SRRs have also increased over the period. The upward trends, in the period 1976-1984, for bladder and malignant neoplasm of kidney and other and unspecified urinary organs for females appear from the recent SRRs to be levelling off. However, the situation is less clear for males. The 1985 SRR for carcinoma-in-situ of the cervix uteri was very much higher than in previous years, which themselves showed an upward trend, and the value for 1986 is even higher. However, interpretation of these SRRs needs to take account of possible improvements in the level of completeness of registration. **Table 1** shows secular trends for other sites also. Care should be taken particularly when interpreting data for sites with small numbers of registrations.

Cancer registrations

Annual registration tables

The diagnosis in all tables is classified according to the Ninth Revision of the *International Classification of Diseases* (ICD).[3]

Table 1 presents standardised registration ratios by sex and site in the 10-year period up to 1986. **Tables 2** to **5**, **7** and **10** show registration numbers or rates by sex and age.

Tables 8 and **11** show standardised registration ratios by sex. **Tables 6, 9** and **12** show directly age standardised rates by sex of newly diagnosed cases of cancer.

Appendix A shows the estimated resident population as at 30 June 1986.

Registrations with residence not stated and residence outside England and Wales are excluded from all tables, except in **Appendix B** where residence outside England and Wales cases are shown.

Appendix C shows cancer incidence to mortality ratios.

As a result of administrative problems experienced in 1985 when the combined Thames Cancer Registry came into operation, there was a shortfall (compared with earlier years) in registrations in the North East Thames region. There was also a shortfall in 1985 of around 10 per cent of registrations for the North Western region because of problems experienced with the processing of one set of data from the Registry.

Survival tables

OPCS registrations since 1971 have been updated (as already described) and the latest survival tables have been published in *Cancer survival 1981 registrations*.[5] Extensive material for England and Wales is given in *Trends in cancer survival in Great Britain*.[6]

Validity of statistics

The validity of cancer registration statistics depends on (1) the completeness of ascertainment and (2) the correctness of the items recorded for each patient registered as suffering from cancer.

Completeness of the national cancer registration data is necessarily dependent on the registration in each regional health authority. In an attempt to compare completeness of ascertainment between RHAs, tables have been published in the past relating the numbers of registrations to the number of deaths from malignant disease. However, because the survival rates in the first few years after diagnosis vary appreciably for different cancers, it is more appropriate to make such a comparison for specific sites of malignancy. For the present report, Appendix C presents cancer incidence to mortality ratios by sex and site.

More precise checks have been carried out by a variety of *ad hoc* studies, using different sources of information to gauge the proportion of patients with malignant disease who were not registered in the regional systems. The results of such studies cannot automatically be applied to the overall coverage of the national scheme, but they do suggest that up to 10 per cent of registrations may be missing from the national data.

The other important aspect of validity of the statistics is the correctness of the items provided for each patient registered with the scheme. OPCS has no direct facility to check such material, but a series of indirect checks have been instituted, such as looking at the percentage of items missing in records submitted from different regions.

The ten most common cancer sites

The ten most common malignant sites registered in England and Wales in 1986 are shown as follows, by sex, with the number of registrations and the percentage that each of the ten sites forms of all sites.

Site description	Number	Per cent*
a) Males		
All sites (ICD 140-208)	103,495	100
Trachea, bronchus and lung	24,365	24
Skin other than melanoma	14,152	14
Prostate	10,180	10
Bladder	6,781	7
Stomach	6,624	6
Colon	6,542	6
Rectum, rectosigmoid junction and anus	5,168	5
Pancreas	2,756	3
Oesophagus	2,591	3
Kidney and other and unspecified urinary organs	1,906	2
Others	22,430	22

b) Females

All sites (ICD 140-208)	102,309	100
Breast	22,757	22
Skin other than melanoma	12,615	12
Trachea, bronchus and lung	9,991	10
Colon	8,234	8
Ovary and other uterine adnexa	4,507	4
Rectum, rectosigmoid junction and anus	4,159	4
Cervix uteri	4,034	4
Stomach	4,029	4
Body of uterus	3,432	3
Pancreas	2,831	3
Others	25,720	25

* The sum of percentages for individual sites may not add to 100 because of rounding.

Cumulative risk of cancer registration

Table A shows the application of a life table method to the presentation of 1986 cancer registration data for males and females over all malignant sites (ICD 140-208). Column 2 of the table shows the number of survivors from a cohort and is based on an England and Wales life table using 1985-1987 mortality data. This is a hypothetical cohort, not a birth cohort, and is dependent entirely on the age-specific death rates prevailing in the years for which it is constructed (an example of the survival calculation is given in *OPCS Monitor* MB1 88/1). Column 4 shows the percentage of this cohort that would be registered with a malignancy in each age-group using 1986 registration rates. The final column shows the percentage of this cohort that would be registered up to and including the particular age-group and is a measure of the risk of registration up to that age.

From the Table it can be seen that 35 per cent of the cohort of males and 33 per cent of the cohort of females would eventually be registered with some form of malignancy. However, registrations would not be equally spread across age-groups. Only 7 per cent of the cohort of males (one fifth of the total) and 9 per cent of the cohort of females (one quarter of the total) would be registered at ages below 60.

Table A Cumulative percentages registered for all sites (ICD 140-208) by sex and age in England and Wales, 1986

Age-group (1)	Survivors from cohort of 10,000 (2)	Cancer registrations rate per 10,000 (3)	Percentage of cohort registered in age-group (4)	Cumulative percentage registered (5)
Males				
0-14	9,875	1.06	0.16	0.16
15-19	9,838	1.66	0.08	0.24
20-24	9,797	2.10	0.10	0.34
25-29	9,759	3.28	0.16	0.50
30-34	9,717	4.17	0.20	0.70
35-39	9,663	6.41	0.31	1.01
40-44	9,583	10.58	0.51	1.52
45-49	9,445	18.78	0.89	2.41
50-54	9,208	34.29	1.58	3.99
55-59	8,797	61.34	2.70	6.69
60-64	8,107	104.89	4.25	10.94
65-69	7,090	152.95	5.42	16.36
70-74	5,709	214.58	6.13	22.49
75-79	4,049	278.60	5.64	28.13
80-84	2,378	325.33	3.87	32.00
85 and over	486	357.40	2.61	34.61
Females				
0-14	9,903	0.88	0.13	0.13
15-19	9,880	1.22	0.06	0.19
20-24	9,864	1.95	0.10	0.29
25-29	9,848	4.12	0.20	0.49
30-34	9,825	8.31	0.41	0.90
35-39	9,790	13.94	0.68	1.58
40-44	9,735	21.40	1.04	2.62
45-49	9,643	31.69	1.53	4.15
50-54	9,490	44.31	2.10	6.25
55-59	9,238	59.67	2.76	9.01
60-64	8,825	80.75	3.56	12.57
65-69	8,204	99.23	4.07	16.64
70-74	7,306	123.29	4.50	21.14
75-79	6,042	144.10	4.35	25.49
80-84	4,389	165.65	3.64	29.13
85 and over	1,270	197.31	3.76	32.89

Definitions

Cancer

For the purposes of the national cancer registration scheme the term 'cancer' includes all malignant neoplasms and the reticuloses, that is conditions listed under site code numbers 140 to 208 of the ICD, Ninth Revision.[3] In addition, all carcinoma in-situ and neoplasms of uncertain behaviour are registered. Benign neoplasms and neoplasms of unspecified nature of bladder and brain, including the pineal and pituitary bodies, are also registered, together with hydatidiform mole.

It should be noted that some cancer registries are not always able to collect complete information about benign, uncertain and unspecified neoplasms and therefore these registration rates are almost certainly underestimates of the true incidence. In particular this should be noted when interpreting regional differences (**Tables 7** to **9**).

Populations

The population figures used to calculate incidence rates given in this volume are the revised mid-year estimates of the population resident in England and Wales. They are based on the 1981 census and use a slightly different definition of residents from the pre-1981 estimates: residents who were outside Great Britain on census night are now included whereas overseas visitors to Great Britain are now excluded. Consequently, the mid 1986 estimates are not directly comparable with those produced for years before 1981.

Appendix A shows the populations for each regional health authority, metropolitan county and predominantly urban and predominantly rural area by sex and age. These population estimates were the latest available at the time of going to print but may have been revised since. Users wishing to check the latest estimates should contact:

Population Estimates Unit
Office of Population Censuses and Surveys
St Catherines House
10 Kingsway
London
WC2B 6JP

Regional health authorities

Cancer registrations are recorded by cancer registries based on the registry or regional health authority area. The tables in this report are presented by administrative RHA of usual residence.

Some regional cancer registry publications present regional statistics based on the number of patients treated in the cancer registry area. Therefore statistics in some regional cancer registry reports may differ from the region of residence analyses shown in this report.

Appendix B shows the redistribution of registrations from the registry area to the RHA of residence. North Thames, South Thames, Mersey and East Anglia RHAs are recipients of the largest number of cancer patients resident outside their boundaries. It should be noted that one cancer registry (Thames) registers cancer patients in all four Thames RHAs.

From 1 April 1982, a single structure of 192 district health authorities replaced the former area health authorities and health districts in England. Certain regional health authorities were also affected by boundary changes. As a result of these and subsequent changes the 1986 RHAs as defined in terms of the new district health authorities were as follows:

Northern	**Yorkshire**
Hartlepool	Hull
North Tees	East Yorkshire
South Tees	Grimsby
East Cumbria	Scunthorpe
South Cumbria	Northallerton
West Cumbria	York
Darlington	Scarborough
Durham	Harrogate
North West Durham	Bradford
South West Durham	Airedale
Northumberland	Calderdale
	Huddersfield
Gateshead	
Newcastle	Dewsbury
North Tyneside	Leeds Western
South Tyneside	Leeds Eastern
Sunderland	Wakefield
	Pontefract

Trent
North Derbyshire
South Derbyshire
Leicestershire
North Lincolnshire
South Lincolnshire
Bassetlaw
Central Nottinghamshire
Nottingham
Barnsley
Doncaster
Rotherham
Sheffield

East Anglian
Cambridge
Peterborough
West Suffolk
East Suffolk
Norwich
Great Yarmouth and
  Waveney
West Norfolk and
  Wisbech
Huntingdon

North West Thames
North Bedfordshire
South Bedfordshire
North Hertfordshire
East Hertfordshire
North West Hertfordshire

South West Hertfordshire
Barnet
Harrow
Hillingdon
Hounslow and Spelthorne
Ealing
Brent
Paddington and North
  Kensington
Riverside

North East Thames
Basildon and Thurrock
Mid Essex
North East Essex
West Essex
Southend
Barking, Havering and
  Brentwood
Hampstead
Bloomsbury
Islington
City and Hackney
Newham

North East Thames - *continued*

Tower Hamlets
Enfield
Harringey

Redbridge
Waltham Forest

South East Thames
Brighton
Eastbourne
Hastings
South East Kent
Canterbury and Thanet

Dartford and Gravesham
Maidstone
Medway
Tunbridge Wells
Bexley

Greenwich
Bromley
West Lambeth
Camberwell
Lewisham and North
  Southwark

South West Thames
North West Surrey
West Surrey and North
  East Hampshire
South West Surrey
Mid Surrey
East Surrey
Chichester
Mid Downs

Worthing
Croydon
Kingston and Esher
Richmond, Twickenham
  and Roehampton
Wandsworth
Merton and Sutton

Wessex
East Dorset
West Dorset
Portsmouth and South
  East Hampshire
Southampton and South
  West Hampshire
Winchester

Wessex - *continued*

Basingstoke and North
  Hampshire
Salisbury
Swindon
Bath
Isle of Wight

Oxford
East Berkshire
West Berkshire
Aylesbury Vale
Wycombe
Milton Keynes
Kettering
Northampton
Oxfordshire

South Western
Bristol and Weston
Frenchay
Southmead
Cornwall and Isles
  of Scilly
Exeter
North Devon

Plymouth
Torbay
Cheltenham and District
Gloucester
Somerset

West Midlands
Bromsgrove and Redditch
Herefordshire
Kidderminster and District
Worcester and District
Shropshire
Mid Staffordshire

North Staffordshire
South East Staffordshire
Rugby
North Warwickshire
South Warwickshire
Central Birmingham
East Birmingham
North Birmingham

West Midlands - *continued*

South Birmingham
West Birmingham
Coventry

Dudley
Sandwell
Solihull
Walsall
Wolverhampton

Mersey
Chester
Crewe
Halton
Macclesfield
Warrington

Liverpool
St Helens and Knowsley
Southport and Formby
South Sefton
Wirral

North Western
Lancaster
Blackpool, Wyre and Fylde
Preston
Blackburn, Hyndburn and
  Ribble Valley
Burnley, Pendle and
  Rossendale
West Lancashire
Chorley and South Ribble
Bolton

Bury
North Manchester
Central Manchester
South Manchester
Oldham
Rochdale

Salford
Stockport
Tameside and Glossop
Trafford
Wigan

In 1986 the district health authorities in Wales were as follows:

Clwyd	Mid Glamorgan
East Dyfed	Powys
Pembrokeshire	South Glamorgan
Gwent	West Glamorgan
Gwynedd	

Predominantly urban and predominantly rural aggregations

In this report the method of tabulating urban and rural statistics is by aggregating county districts. Studies by Webber and Craig[7,8] have shown that districts which are at the rural end of the range of variations can be identified.

Tables 10 to **12** use the metropolitan counties, the aggregated predominantly rural areas and the remainder (called predominantly urban). The total populations of these areas are shown in **Appendix A**.

The metropolitan county, predominantly rural and predominantly urban areas relate to the following aggregations:

Metropolitan counties

Greater London, Greater Manchester, Merseyside, South Yorkshire, Tyne and Wear, West Midlands, West Yorkshire.

Predominantly urban areas

Remainder of England and Wales, excluding predominantly rural areas and metropolitan counties.

Predominantly rural areas

Alnwick
Arfon (Gwynedd)
Ashford
Aylesbury Vale
Babergh (Suffolk)
Berwick-upon-Tweed
Boothferry
  (Humberside)
Boston
Braintree
Breckland (Norfolk)
Brecknock (Powys)
Bridgnorth
Broadland (Norfolk)
Caradon
Carmarthen
Carrick (Cornwall)
Chichester
Colchester
Cotswold
Craven
  (North Yorkshire)
Daventry
Dinefwr (Dyfed)
Dwyfor (Gwynedd)
East Cambridgeshire
East Hampshire
East Hertfordshire
East Lindsey
East Yorkshire
Eden (Cumbria)
Fenland
  (Cambridgeshire)
Forest Heath
Ceredigion
Cherwell (Oxfordshire)
Chester
Glanford
  (Humberside)
Glyndwr
  (Clwyd)
Hambleton
  (North Yorkshire)
Holderness
Kennet (Wiltshire)
Kerrier (Cornwall)
Leominster
Maidstone
Maldon (Essex)
Malvern Hills
Meirionnydd
  (Gwynedd)
Melton
  (Leicestershire)
Mendip
Mid Devon
Mid Suffolk
Monmouth
Montgomery
Newbury
North Bedfordshire
North Cornwall
North Devon
North Dorset
North Kesteven
North Norfolk
North Shropshire
North Wiltshire
Oswestry
Penwith (Cornwall)
Preseli (Dyfed)
Purbeck (Dorset)
Radnor (Powys)
Restormel (Cornwall)
Richmondshire
  (North Yorkshire)
Rutland
Ryedale
  (North Yorkshire)
(Suffolk)
Forest of Dean
Salisbury
Scilly Isles
Sedgemoor (Somerset)
Selby
Shrewsbury and Atcham
South Cambridgeshire
South Hams (Devon)
South Herefordshire
South Holland
South Kesteven
South Lakeland
South Norfolk
South Northamptonshire
South Oxfordshire
South Pembrokeshire
South Shropshire
St Edmundsbury
  (Suffolk)
Stratford-on-Avon
Suffolk Coastal
Teesdale
Test Valley
Tewkesbury
Torridge (Devon)
Tunbridge Wells
Tynedale
  (Northumberland)
Uttlesford (Essex)
Vale of Glamorgan
Vale of White Horse
  (Oxfordshire)
Waveney (Suffolk)
West Derbyshire
West Devon
West Dorset
West Lindsey
West Norfolk
West Oxfordshire
West Somerset
Winchester
Wychavon (Hereford
  and Worcester)
Yeovil
Ynys Mon (Gwynedd)

7

Standardised registration ratio (SRR)

The incidence of cancer varies greatly with age. The SRR is an index which enables ready comparison of incidence rates in populations with different age structures. It is calculated by denoting one set of age-specific rates as the standard. These are then applied to each of several index populations of known age structure to show how many registrations would have been expected in these index populations had they, at each age, experienced the cancer incidence of the standard population. The 'expected' incidence so found is then compared with the observed, their ratio being multiplied by 100 to give an index in which 100 is the value for the standard population. **Table 1** shows, for each cancer, trends in registration from 1977 to 1986. Experience in 1979 is taken as the standard. The SRRs shown in this table may be different from those shown in *Series MB1* prior to 1982 because they have been recalculated to take account of the following changes:

a. revised population estimates based on the 1981 Census (see page 5).

b. the addition of late registrations to the national dataset.

c. the effect of the above on the base year 1979.

Calculations for 1986 are based on nineteen age-groups; for instance the SRR for cancer of the stomach was calculated as:

$$SRR = \frac{100 \times \text{registration of cancer of the stomach in 1986 aged under 75}}{\sum_{\text{age-group}} \left[\begin{array}{l} \text{Population at each age, 1986} \times \\ \text{registration rate for cancer of} \\ \text{the stomach for that age in 1979} \end{array} \right]}$$

for each sex separately.

Table 8 shows the 1986 SRRs in RHAs of residence. For each cancer, the registration rates in England and Wales are taken as the standards (with the sexes considered separately). For example, the SRR for cancer of the stomach in the Northern RHA was calculated as

$$SRR = \frac{100 \times \text{registration of cancer of the stomach in Northern RHA}}{\sum_{\text{age-group}} \left[\begin{array}{l} \text{population at each age, Northern RHA} \times \\ \text{registration rate for cancer of the stomach} \\ \text{for that age, England and Wales} \end{array} \right]}$$

Symbols and conventions used

-   nil
..   not available
:   not appropriate
nos   not otherwise specified
nec   not elsewhere classified

In the printed tables, rates calculated from less than 20 registrations are distinguished by italic type as a warning to the user that their reliability as a measure may be affected by the small number of registrations. For technical reasons it is not possible to italicise figures appearing on fiche. Readers are advised to refer to other tables to determine the number of registrations upon which rates are based.

Further information

Users may wish to know that special tabulations are available to order (subject to confidentiality thresholds) and on repayment. Such requests or enquiries should be made to:

Cancer Registration Section
Office of Population Censuses and Surveys
Segensworth Road
Titchfield
Fareham
Hants
PO15 5RR

Acknowledgement

The continuing co-operation of regional cancer registries in England and Wales, in support of the publication of these statistics is gratefully acknowledged.

References

1. *Report of the Advisory Committee on Cancer Registration, 1980*: Cancer registration in the 1980s. Series MB1 no.6. HMSO (1981).

2. *A Review of the National Cancer Registration System in England and Wales*. Series MB1 no. 17. HMSO (1990).

3. *International Classification of Diseases, Injuries and Causes of Death,* Ninth Revision. WHO, Geneva (1977).

4. *Cancer registration surveillance, 1968-1978.* OPCS (1983).

5. Cancer survival 1981 registrations *OPCS Monitor* MB1 88/1, OPCS (1988).

6. *Trends in cancer survival in Great Britain.* Cancer Research Campaign (1982).

7. Webber R and Craig J. Which local authorities are alike? *Population Trends 5.* HMSO (1976).

8. Craig J. Urban and rural local authorities. *Population Trends 8.* HMSO (1977).

Series MB1 no. 19 Table 1

Table 1 Standardised registration ratios for persons aged under 75 (base year 1979): sex and site, 1977 - 1986   England and Wales

ICD (9th Revision) number	Site description	Sex	1977	1978	1979	1980	1981	1982	1983	1984	1985**	1986
140-208	**All malignant neoplasms**	M	**103**	**100**	**100**	**99**	**100**	**100**	**100**	**101**	**99**	**99**
		F	**102**	**102**	**100**	**101**	**103**	**104**	**104**	**105**	**102**	**105**
140	Malignant neoplasm of lip	M	91	66	100	108	83	83	65	64	64	65
		F	97	80	100	107	117	92	90	109	89	79
141	Malignant neoplasm of tongue	M	96	86	100	101	99	116	97	115	92	93
		F	93	81	100	92	97	99	105	112	87	84
142	Malignant neoplasm of major salivary glands	M	121	114	100	87	80	89	80	90	91	80
		F	135	112	100	76	91	72	81	83	74	84
143	Malignant neoplasm of gum	M	..	..	100	97	100	81	71	104	60	100
		F	..	..	100	75	137	90	94	88	80	64
144	Malignant neoplasm of floor of mouth	M	111	113	100	98	133	116	117	122	109	124
		F	86	106	100	105	83	111	110	117	107	86
145	Malignant neoplasm of other and unspecified parts of mouth	M	103	94	100	99	92	103	104	111	89	96
		F	98	119	100	83	106	119	127	110	112	117
146	Malignant neoplasm of oropharynx	M	90*	103*	100	106	100	115	106	98	84	92
		F	128*	122*	100	104	122	127	105	117	107	113
147	Malignant neoplasm of nasopharynx	M	..	..	100	127	117	96	123	120	86	92
		F	..	..	100	126	108	98	67	97	98	85
148	Malignant neoplasm of hypopharynx	M	93	79	100	106	99	86	115	110	116	102
		F	94	114	100	94	105	93	85	83	82	66
149	Malignant neoplasm of other and ill-defined sites within the lip, oral cavity and pharynx	M	105	100	100	106	109	120	113	110	100	104
		F	129	121	100	117	109	108	115	93	106	76
150	Malignant neoplasm of oesophagus	M	108	115	100	108	112	122	115	124	113	122
		F	103	111	100	100	107	108	112	116	101	101
151	Malignant neoplasm of stomach	M	106	104	100	102	98	95	96	91	88	88
		F	107	104	100	91	92	88	87	88	80	76
152	Malignant neoplasm of small intestine, including duodenum	M	110	99	100	94	90	92	105	105	109	92
		F	94	101	100	79	84	72	84	93	78	83
153	Malignant neoplasm of colon	M	102	100	100	99	102	105	104	107	100	100
		F	105	103	100	96	104	102	101	100	95	97
154	Malignant neoplasm of rectum, rectosigmoid junction and anus	M	98	95	100	97	98	99	97	101	98	95
		F	103	107	100	103	102	106	107	102	92	93
155	Malignant neoplasm of liver and intrahepatic bile-ducts	M	..	..	100	96	93	95	101	104	99	96
		F	..	..	100	105	110	112	113	120	110	105
156	Malignant neoplasm of gallbladder and extrahepatic bile ducts	M	115	116	100	100	95	103	93	97	92	97
		F	106	101	100	101	96	90	92	97	92	89
157	Malignant neoplasm of pancreas	M	97	99	100	92	96	93	90	93	86	83
		F	97	98	100	92	92	102	96	96	95	95
158	Malignant neoplasm of retroperitoneum and peritoneum	M	83	105	100	79	81	84	100	80	83	76
		F	95	91	100	90	95	96	79	97	76	67
159	Malignant neoplasm of other and ill-defined sites within the digestive organs and peritoneum	M	..	..	100	110	103	102	91	96	117	109
		F	..	..	100	97	96	96	108	95	117	116
160	Malignant neoplasm of nasal cavities, middle ear and accessory sinuses	M	..	..	100	91	85	85	92	78	81	90
		F	..	..	100	69	87	101	77	93	91	92

* Results published in *Mortality statistics* (Series DH1 No.10) show that the changes from the 8th to 9th Revision of the ICD produce losses or gains of registrations for some sites. Where these changes are of the order of 10 to 20 per cent a warning(*) has been entered against the 1976-78 SRRs. Where larger changes have occurred only 1979-85 SRRs are shown.
† For years shown, SRRs are calculated from the revised mid year estimates of population based on the 1981 Census. See pages 5 and 8.
**SRRs for persons of all ages.

9

Table 1 Series MB1 no. 19

Table 1 Standardised registration ratios - *continued*

ICD (9th Revision) number	Site description		Year of registration†									
			1977	1978	1979	1980	1981	1982	1983	1984	1985**	1986
161	Malignant neoplasm of larynx	M	103	103	100	103	102	106	99	105	96	99
		F	107	109	100	103	103	101	97	98	93	102
162	Malignant neoplasm of trachea, bronchus and lung	M	106	100	100	97	95	95	92	91	88	84
		F	94	97	100	101	108	112	112	115	115	117
163	Malignant neoplasm of pleura	M	..	..	100	112	101	115	128	146	148	191
		F	..	..	100	75	79	75	75	83	70	85
164	Malignant neoplasm of thymus, heart and mediastinum	M	..	..	100	112	147	113	154	123	153	120
		F	..	..	100	125	75	121	103	134	100	102
165	Malignant neoplasm of other and ill-defined sites within the respiratory system and intrathoracic organs	M	..	..	100	12	53	63	13	13	47	*41*
		F	..	..	100	25	50	13	26	26	13	*13*
170	Malignant neoplasm of bone and articular cartilage	M	97*	94*	100	92	115	77	85	86	93	87
		F	186*	96*	100	94	119	84	82	90	111	106
171	Malignant neoplasm of connective and other soft tissue	M	189*	91*	100	90	96	88	93	91	87	96
		F	84*	89*	100	105	104	78	89	85	98	99
172	Malignant melanoma of skin	M	90	95	100	107	115	114	121	118	134	142
		F	93	95	100	104	111	116	121	120	135	141
173	Other malignant neoplasm of skin	M	102*	104*	100	102	105	100	102	104	114	127
		F	101*	104*	100	101	107	103	108	110	111	129
174	Malignant neoplasm of female breast	F	105	106	100	103	102	105	102	102	102	105
175	Malignant neoplasm of male breast	M	123	129	100	95	103	98	92	106	98	85
179	Malignant neoplasm of uterus, part unspecified	F	..	..	100	102	95	98	119	90	88	84
180	Malignant neoplasm of cervix uteri	F	103	99	100	101	103	101	100	105	101	102
181	Malignant neoplasm of placenta	F	157	106	100	78	67	70	66	59	47	*56*
182	Malignant neoplasm of body of uterus	F	..	..	100	101	100	100	96	96	96	98
183	Malignant neoplasm of ovary and other uterine adnexa	F	104	101	100	102	102	102	104	103	100	103
184	Malignant neoplasm of other and unspecified female genital organs	F	106	101	100	100	91	96	85	106	92	94
185	Malignant neoplasm of prostate	M	101	94	100	102	104	107	111	117	103	108
186	Malignant neoplasm of testis	M	105	113	100	111	120	116	111	122	116	127
187	Malignant neoplasm of penis and other male genital organs	M	95*	87*	100	116	101	96	91	91	99	93
188	Malignant neoplasm of bladder	M	100	100	100	101	104	102	106	108	103	100
		F	96	94	100	97	108	103	107	113	104	111
189	Malignant neoplasm of kidney and other and unspecified urinary organs	M	103	100	100	102	107	114	112	123	112	110
		F	97	99	100	102	104	111	112	119	113	115
190	Malignant neoplasm of eye	M	107	115	100	86	101	90	109	102	107	114
		F	122	115	100	100	118	117	104	126	97	96
191	Malignant neoplasm of brain	M	94	90	100	97	104	97	102	103	105	105
		F	91	88	100	97	103	97	104	109	108	103

* Results published in *Mortality statistics* (Series DH1 No.10) show that the changes from the 8th to 9th Revision of the ICD produce losses or gains of registrations for some sites. Where these changes are of the order of 10 to 20 per cent a warning(*) has been entered against the 1976-78 SRRs. Where larger changes have occurred only 1979-85 SRRs are shown.
† For years shown, SRRs are calculated from the revised mid year estimates of population based on the 1981 Census. See pages 5 and 8.
**SRRs for persons of all ages

Table 1 Standardised registration ratios - *continued*

ICD (9th Revision) number	Site description		1977	1978	1979	1980	1981	1982	1983	1984	1985**	1986
192	Malignant neoplasm of other and unspecified parts of nervous system	M	..	..	100	71	97	71	77	86	89	69
		F	..	..	100	127	134	100	170	142	92	83
193	Malignant neoplasm of thyroid gland	M	103	96	100	115	114	108	117	114	111	112
		F	117	99	100	112	107	118	112	103	82	91
194	Malignant neoplasm of other endocrine glands and related structures	M	..	..	100	106	85	82	105	92	87	63
		F	..	..	100	83	93	61	82	88	57	69
195	Malignant neoplasm of other and ill-defined sites	M	..	..	100	96	95	104	110	93	69	57
		F	..	..	100	81	82	97	93	71	58	63
196	Secondary and unspecified malignant neoplasm of lymph nodes	M	116	109	100	107	106	121	99	100	107	94
		F	106	118	100	115	114	121	89	92	117	114
197	Secondary malignant neoplasm of respiratory and digestive systems	M	100	106	100	96	117	116	89	115	126	133
		F	121	109	100	111	127	128	109	129	137	144
198	Secondary malignant neoplasm of other specified sites	M	94	110	100	97	115	122	99	114	125	112
		F	97	100	100	102	121	121	106	124	129	121
199	Malignant neoplasm without specification of site	M	..	..	100	101	88	113	136	129	113	122
		F	..	..	100	100	85	108	130	111	112	110
200	Lymphosarcoma and reticulosarcoma	M	147	133	100	96	90	72	63	52	45	44
		F	153	131	100	95	88	74	69	51	47	39
201	Hodgkin's disease	M	117	116	100	103	101	95	95	87	86	88
		F	109	100	100	110	101	92	96	97	92	87
202	Other malignant neoplasm of lymphoid and histiocytic tissue	M	..	..	100	102	105	116	132	147	162	174
		F	..	..	100	106	115	128	144	152	176	186
203	Multiple myeloma and immunoproliferative neoplasms	M	103	103	100	92	98	89	104	99	108	110
		F	114	107	100	104	100	106	98	107	112	102
204-208	All leukaemias	M	..	..	100	93	97	92	97	98	96	88
		F	..	..	100	96	99	95	109	108	99	94
204	Lymphoid leukaemia	M	100	102	100	96	98	82	92	89	96	88
		F	119	112	100	110	109	101	112	109	111	100
205	Myeloid leukaemia	M	104	96	100	86	92	92	84	91	99	93
		F	111	101	100	85	93	86	90	90	94	96
206	Monocytic leukaemia	M	173*	144*	100	121	147	116	114	90	83	64
		F	134*	131*	100	100	52	85	103	89	81	94
207	Other specified leukaemia	M	..	..	100	86	76	78	63	66	51	47
		F	..	..	100	122	95	88	60	77	82	66
208	Leukaemia of unspecified cell type	M	..	..	100	117	118	158	216	213	98	80
		F	..	..	100	96	113	138	253	248	88	68
223.3	Benign neoplasm of bladder	M	..	..	100	91	108	80	78	52	46	24
		F	..	..	100	97	112	129	97	79	47	*31*
225	Benign neoplasm of brain and other parts of nervous system	M	..	..	100	108	113	114	98	127	124	114
		F	..	..	100	98	102	103	109	112	119	108
227.3	Benign neoplasm of pituitary gland and craniopharyngeal duct	M	..	..	100	94	96	109	113	127	129	112
		F	..	..	100	97	108	114	134	128	121	114
227.4	Benign neoplasm of pineal gland≠	M	..	..	-	-	-	-	-	-	-	-
		F	..	..	-	-	-	-	-	-	-	-

* Results published in *Mortality statistics* (Series DH1 No.10) show that the changes from the 8th to 9th Revision of the ICD produce losses or gains of registrations for some sites. Where these changes are of the order of 10 to 20 per cent a warning(*) has been entered against the 1976-78 SRRs. Where larger changes have occurred only 1979-85 SRRs are shown.
† For years shown, SRRs are calculated from the revised mid year estimates of population based on the 1981 Census. See pages 5 and 8.
≠ SRRs are not shown for ICD 227.4, because there were no registrations except in 1983.
**SRRs for persons of all ages.

Table 1 Standardised registration ratios - *continued*

ICD (9th Revision) number	Site description		1977	1978	1979	1980	1981	1982	1983	1984	1985**	1986
230	Carcinoma in situ of digestive organs	M	..	..	100	126	120	94	93	90	135	133
		F	..	..	100	60	70	82	71	82	113	98
231	Carcinoma in situ of respiratory systems	M	..	..	100	122	140	137	129	151	159	149
		F	..	..	100	77	111	107	113	128	166	204
232	Carcinoma in situ of skin	M	..	..	100	113	133	127	142	142	171	212
		F	..	..	100	118	137	153	158	179	208	238
233	Carcinoma in situ of breast and genitourinary system	M	..	..	100	103	120	118	134	148	190	203
		F	..	..	100	107	122	119	118	179	234	265
233.1	Carcinoma in situ of cervix uteri	F	95	93	100	108	126	128	127	196	259	296
234	Carcinoma in situ of other and unspecified sites	M	..	..	100	200	300	172	310	107	93	*117*
		F	..	..	100	63	71	143	154	68	38	*56*
235	Neoplasm of uncertain behaviour of digestive and respiratory systems	M	..	..	100	114	119	102	110	120	109	102
		F	..	..	100	116	114	128	139	143	146	146
236	Neoplasm of uncertain behaviour of genitourinary organs	M	..	..	100	101	72	88	79	81	49	38
		F	..	..	100	103	111	212	431	155	138	166
237	Neoplasm of uncertain behaviour of endocrine glands and nervous system	M	..	..	100	78	63	60	70	68	72	70
		F	..	..	100	89	80	61	81	89	69	77
238	Neoplasm of uncertain behaviour of other and unspecified sites and tissues	M	..	..	100	120	110	126	118	126	115	117
		F	..	..	100	101	112	120	118	135	140	143
239.4	Neoplasm of unspecified nature of bladder	M	..	..	100	126	120	102	59	60	78	77
		F	..	..	100	113	90	77	65	36	82	78
239.6	Neoplasm of unspecified nature of brain	M	..	..	100	105	84	123	91	87	82	80
		F	..	..	100	100	82	119	99	96	95	93
239.7	Neoplasm of unspecified nature of other parts of nervous system and pituitary gland only	M	..	..	100	100	113	276	145	199	184	194
		F	..	..	100	131	96	70	102	102	62	90
630	Hydatidiform mole	F	..	..	100	95	113	125	140	128	92	90

* Results published in *Mortality statistics* (Series DH1 No.10) show that the changes from the 8th to 9th Revision of the ICD produce losses or gains of registrations for some sites. Where these changes are of the order of 10 to 20 per cent a warning(*) has been entered against the 1976-78 SRRs. Where larger changes have occurred only 1979-85 SRRs are shown.
† For years shown, SRRs are calculated from the revised mid year estimates of population based on the 1981 Census. See pages 5 and 8.
**SRRs for persons of all ages

Table 2 Series MB1 no. 19

Table 2 Registrations of newly diagnosed cases of cancer: sex, site and age, 1986

ICD (9th Revision) number	Site description		All ages	Under 1	1-4	5-9	10-14	15-19	20-24	25-29	30-34	35-39
	All registrations	M	106,605	49	195	150	168	369	491	669	746	1,268
		F	121,186	56	153	112	134	473	1,960	4,062	4,773	5,505
140-208	All malignant neoplasms	M	103,495	44	185	132	154	332	447	615	702	1,186
		F	102,309	48	140	102	113	232	404	761	1,378	2,578
140	Malignant neoplasm of lip	M	198	-	-	-	-	1	-	1	-	3
		F	47	-	-	-	-	-	-	-	-	1
141	Malignant neoplasm of tongue	M	328	-	-	-	-	1	1	1	5	3
		F	213	-	-	-	-	-	2	-	1	7
142	Malignant neoplasm of major salivary glands	M	159	-	-	-	2	1	3	2	4	6
		F	154	-	-	-	1	-	1	1	5	4
143	Malignant neoplasm of gum	M	75	-	-	-	-	-	-	-	-	1
		F	45	-	-	-	-	-	-	-	-	1
144	Malignant neoplasm of floor of mouth	M	214	-	-	-	-	-	-	-	-	4
		F	58	-	-	-	-	-	-	-	-	-
145	Malignant neoplasm of other and unspecified parts of mouth	M	199	-	-	-	1	1	-	2	1	2
		F	139	-	-	-	-	-	-	1	1	2
146	Malignant neoplasm of oropharynx	M	212	-	-	1	-	-	-	-	-	3
		F	101	-	-	-	-	-	1	-	3	2
147	Malignant neoplasm of nasopharynx	M	109	-	-	1	1	2	1	2	2	3
		F	61	-	-	1	-	3	2	4	-	6
148	Malignant neoplasm of hypopharynx	M	207	-	-	-	-	-	1	-	-	-
		F	135	-	-	-	-	-	-	-	-	1
149	Malignant neoplasm of other and ill-defined sites within the lip, oral cavity and pharynx	M	90	-	-	-	-	-	1	-	-	2
		F	43	-	-	-	-	-	-	-	-	3
150	Malignant neoplasm of oesophagus	M	2,591	-	-	-	-	-	1	1	7	21
		F	1,812	-	-	-	-	-	-	-	1	6
151	Malignant neoplasm of stomach	M	6,624	-	-	-	-	1	1	10	9	39
		F	4,029	-	-	-	-	-	2	5	9	18
152	Malignant neoplasm of small intestine, including duodenum	M	153	-	1	-	-	1	-	1	2	3
		F	160	-	-	-	-	-	-	-	3	2
153	Malignant neoplasm of colon	M	6,542	-	-	-	-	3	5	11	20	61
		F	8,234	-	-	-	-	2	4	9	23	62
154	Malignant neoplasm of rectum, rectosigmoid junction and anus	M	5,168	-	-	1	-	1	5	9	14	36
		F	4,159	1	-	-	-	-	1	4	12	25
155	Malignant neoplasm of liver and intrahepatic bile ducts	M	599	1	3	1	1	1	-	5	7	9
		F	389	1	1	3	2	-	4	-	5	5
156	Malignant neoplasm of gallbladder and extrahepatic bile ducts	M	477	-	-	-	-	1	-	1	-	2
		F	695	-	-	-	-	-	-	-	2	5
157	Malignant neoplasm of pancreas	M	2,756	1	-	-	1	-	-	5	7	15
		F	2,831	-	-	-	1	1	-	2	4	14
158	Malignant neoplasm of retroperitoneum and peritoneum	M	105	-	-	-	-	1	5	1	1	1
		F	122	-	1	-	-	1	1	1	4	1
159	Malignant neoplasm of other and ill-defined sites within the digestive organs and peritoneum	M	170	-	-	-	-	-	1	-	-	2
		F	194	-	-	-	-	-	1	1	-	1
160	Malignant neoplasm of nasal cavities, middle ear and accessory sinuses	M	214	-	-	2	1	3	1	2	-	6
		F	154	-	-	-	-	1	-	1	2	5
161	Malignant neoplasm of larynx	M	1,465	-	-	-	-	-	-	1	1	8
		F	319	-	-	-	-	-	1	2	3	1

England and Wales

40-44	45-49	50-54	55-59	60-64	65-69	70-74	75-79	80-84	85 and over		Site description	ICD (9th Revision) number
1,795	2,762	4,757	8,459	14,027	16,842	19,763	17,819	10,813	5,463	M	All registrations	
5,198	5,478	6,635	8,841	12,152	13,304	15,557	15,151	11,754	9,888	F		
1,686	2,618	4,574	8,151	13,629	16,388	19,251	17,438	10,603	5,360	M	All malignant neoplasms	140-208
3,360	4,380	5,905	8,199	11,427	12,695	14,920	14,611	11,407	9,649	F		
5	8	10	11	26	41	26	38	17	11	M	Malignant neoplasm of lip	140
1	-	-	1	1	6	12	7	12	6	F		
15	24	31	40	51	48	36	45	18	9	M	Malignant neoplasm of tongue	141
7	7	12	15	19	25	32	32	31	23	F		
4	9	11	11	9	22	27	20	18	10	M	Malignant neoplasm of major salivary glands	142
13	8	9	10	10	17	22	17	20	16	F		
2	2	10	9	8	12	10	15	3	3	M	Malignant neoplasm of gum	143
1	1	2	2	9	5	8	2	7	7	F		
4	21	21	34	43	34	26	16	5	6	M	Malignant neoplasm of floor of mouth	144
-	2	4	5	14	6	7	7	8	5	F		
6	10	13	27	35	31	25	20	15	10	M	Malignant neoplasm of other and unspecified parts of mouth	145
1	7	14	9	16	24	21	23	13	7	F		
11	14	19	29	35	34	24	23	12	7	M	Malignant neoplasm of oropharynx	146
5	4	7	9	19	16	13	8	8	6	F		
5	12	9	11	18	15	11	7	8	1	M	Malignant neoplasm of nasopharynx	147
1	1	7	4	8	7	5	6	4	2	F		
3	11	18	26	45	27	36	22	11	7	M	Malignant neoplasm of hypopharynx	148
2	4	11	11	11	27	26	20	13	9	F		
1	5	5	10	18	16	14	9	5	4	M	Malignant neoplasm of other and ill-defined sites within the lip, oral cavity and pharynx	149
-	1	5	3	5	4	9	7	2	4	F		
29	73	124	239	367	431	484	421	260	133	M	Malignant neoplasm of oesophagus	150
14	29	43	119	163	224	299	353	294	267	F		
57	130	244	511	834	1,070	1,295	1,261	777	385	M	Malignant neoplasm of stomach	151
32	52	95	145	316	417	641	839	767	691	F		
3	10	13	18	24	20	19	19	12	7	M	Malignant neoplasm of small intestine, including duodenum	152
2	3	10	14	27	13	27	27	21	11	F		
92	150	277	519	794	982	1,210	1,204	788	426	M	Malignant neoplasm of colon	153
108	168	331	515	822	934	1,252	1,497	1,301	1,206	F		
84	128	257	431	731	826	971	904	521	249	M	Malignant neoplasm of rectum, rectosigmoid junction and anus	154
55	99	164	286	430	513	680	713	582	594	F		
14	18	40	48	83	107	110	86	44	21	M	Malignant neoplasm of liver and intrahepatic bile ducts	155
3	7	11	27	42	45	60	66	50	57	F		
5	15	22	35	62	82	86	85	50	31	M	Malignant neoplasm of gallbladder and extrahepatic bile ducts	156
10	12	21	50	51	73	125	139	114	93	F		
35	61	123	220	388	470	522	479	271	158	M	Malignant neoplasm of pancreas	157
17	36	83	136	253	369	494	579	443	399	F		
5	6	5	8	25	18	11	12	4	2	M	Malignant neoplasm of retroperitoneum and peritoneum	158
3	10	7	7	19	15	17	18	12	5	F		
3	1	6	13	20	35	24	31	23	11	M	Malignant neoplasm of other and ill-defined sites within the digestive organs and peritoneum	159
-	1	6	6	15	13	31	33	37	49	F		
4	9	14	22	30	29	40	28	14	9	M	Malignant neoplasm of nasal cavities, middle ear and accessory sinuses	160
1	7	10	9	18	18	17	23	22	20	F		
31	49	102	178	282	263	264	153	88	45	M	Malignant neoplasm of larynx	161
9	14	18	30	68	53	48	35	16	21	F		

Table 2 Series MB1 no. 19

Table 2 Registrations - *continued*

ICD (9th Revision) number	Site description		All ages	Age-group								
				Under 1	1-4	5-9	10-14	15-19	20-24	25-29	30-34	35-39
162	Malignant neoplasm of trachea, bronchus and lung	M F	24,365 9,991	- -	- -	1 -	- 1	1 1	5 1	8 12	27 14	81 60
163	Malignant neoplasm of pleura	M F	504 97	- -	- -	- -	- -	- -	- -	- -	2 -	7 3
164	Malignant neoplasm of thymus, heart and mediastinum	M F	69 51	- 1	1 -	- 1	1 -	3 -	4 -	4 2	5 2	3 3
165	Malignant neoplasm of other and ill-defined sites within the respiratory system and intrathoracic organs	M F	7 1	- -	- -	- -	- -	- -	- -	- -	- -	- -
170	Malignant neoplasm of bone and articular cartilage	M F	221 216	2 2	1 4	6 6	11 17	32 18	19 21	5 5	3 6	9 9
171	Malignant neoplasm of connective and other soft tissue	M F	453 423	1 6	6 9	7 3	8 9	16 13	16 10	13 11	13 12	26 22
172	Malignant melanoma of skin	M F	989 1,813	- -	1 -	1 1	4 4	8 20	26 43	48 83	42 97	70 134
173	Other malignant neoplasm of skin	M F	14,152 12,615	- 2	- 2	- 1	5 4	9 9	10 24	40 36	85 105	183 208
174	Malignant neoplasm of female breast	F	22,757	1	-	-	2	3	19	122	378	983
175	Malignant neoplasm of male breast	M	155	-	-	-	-	-	-	1	2	3
179	Malignant neoplasm of uterus, part unspecified	F	380	-	-	-	-	-	-	-	6	8
180	Malignant neoplasm of cervix uteri	F	4,034	-	-	-	1	-	42	228	371	487
181	Malignant neoplasm of placenta	F	11	-	-	-	-	1	1	4	3	1
182	Malignant neoplasm of body of uterus	F	3,432	-	-	-	-	1	1	6	13	35
183	Malignant neoplasm of ovary and other uterine adnexa	F	4,507	-	3	-	5	16	32	35	61	114
184	Malignant neoplasm of other and unspecified female genital organs	F	976	-	-	-	-	-	3	10	15	15
185	Malignant neoplasm of prostate	M	10,180	-	-	-	-	-	1	2	-	2
186	Malignant neoplasm of testis	M	1,022	4	9	-	-	44	123	193	171	161
187	Malignant neoplasm of penis and other male genital organs	M	316	-	-	-	-	1	1	2	3	7
188	Malignant neoplasm of bladder	M F	6,781 2,810	- 1	- -	1 -	1 -	1 2	12 3	12 4	31 5	45 16
189	Malignant neoplasm of kidney and other and unspecified urinary organs	M F	1,906 1,185	3 2	15 18	6 10	- -	1 -	4 2	9 6	8 8	37 21
190	Malignant neoplasm of eye	M F	186 155	10 6	7 6	1 -	- -	1 -	3 3	2 -	3 5	6 6
191	Malignant neoplasm of brain	M F	1,520 1,104	3 4	35 17	23 31	31 19	21 26	31 29	39 23	41 28	92 56
192	Malignant neoplasm of other and unspecified parts of nervous system	M F	51 53	1 2	5 5	3 2	3 5	3 2	1 -	6 -	1 3	3 4
193	Malignant neoplasm of thyroid gland	M F	213 521	- -	- -	- -	2 3	6 9	3 29	6 33	13 29	7 43

40-44	45-49	50-54	55-59	60-64	65-69	70-74	75-79	80-84	85 and over		Site description	ICD (9th Revision) number
185	455	866	2,024	3,672	4,449	5,022	4,195	2,347	1,027	M	Malignant neoplasm of trachea, bronchus and lung	162
99	208	391	850	1,527	1,806	1,933	1,498	989	601	F		
20	15	41	65	97	94	74	49	33	7	M	Malignant neoplasm of pleura	163
4	1	3	10	19	17	13	12	11	4	F		
1	2	4	10	11	2	10	5	3	-	M	Malignant neoplasm of thymus, heart and mediastinum	164
3	1	6	6	2	8	5	6	2	3	F		
-	-	2	-	1	-	2	1	-	1	M	Malignant neoplasm of other and ill-defined sites within the respiratory system and intrathoracic organs	165
-	-	-	-	-	1	-	-	-	-	F		
11	8	13	18	24	20	18	11	6	4	M	Malignant neoplasm of bone and articular cartilage	170
8	5	11	12	12	16	21	17	14	12	F		
31	16	31	38	52	44	50	48	27	10	M	Malignant neoplasm of connective and other soft tissue	171
16	18	34	35	33	36	44	45	29	38	F		
77	78	100	85	128	109	76	75	38	23	M	Malignant melanoma of skin	172
166	135	155	152	180	194	165	134	86	64	F		
283	429	779	1,202	1,940	2,231	2,538	2,279	1,373	766	M	Other malignant neoplasm of skin	173
286	399	514	787	1,221	1,531	2,011	2,151	1,804	1,520	F		
1,480	1,891	2,058	2,304	2,800	2,618	2,678	2,326	1,659	1,435	F	Malignant neoplasm of female breast	174
5	9	11	13	20	18	26	23	12	12	M	Malignant neoplasm of male breast	175
6	13	30	35	49	48	52	54	29	50	F	Malignant neoplasm of uterus, part unspecified	179
366	337	278	319	435	386	310	232	127	115	F	Malignant neoplasm of cervix uteri	180
1	-	-	-	-	-	-	-	-	-	F	Malignant neoplasm of placenta	181
66	148	328	517	495	481	493	398	269	181	F	Malignant neoplasm of body of uterus	182
205	268	411	557	559	602	608	493	322	216	F	Malignant neoplasm of ovary and other uterine adnexa	183
13	14	40	45	73	93	165	180	161	149	F	Malignant neoplasm of other and unspecified female genital organs	184
11	22	96	344	839	1,491	2,327	2,417	1,729	899	M	Malignant neoplasm of prostate	185
122	58	46	27	22	11	14	10	5	2	M	Malignant neoplasm of testis	186
9	12	16	24	29	41	53	66	30	22	M	Malignant neoplasm of penis and other male genital organs	187
76	159	290	539	926	1,091	1,334	1,222	694	347	M	Malignant neoplasm of bladder	188
24	51	114	184	310	379	509	483	396	329	F		
44	81	168	203	283	312	294	272	121	45	M	Malignant neoplasm of kidney and other and unspecified urinary organs	189
31	48	65	93	148	162	203	168	118	82	F		
7	13	14	17	22	27	20	24	7	2	M	Malignant neoplasm of eye	190
4	6	10	18	21	11	16	25	10	8	F		
86	125	132	162	218	229	139	73	28	12	M	Malignant neoplasm of brain	191
59	65	79	113	155	157	116	81	31	15	F		
-	4	3	2	6	3	4	3	-	-	M	Malignant neoplasm of other and unspecified parts of nervous system	192
4	2	6	5	2	6	4	-	1	-	F		
10	10	16	28	23	28	21	20	14	6	M	Malignant neoplasm of thyroid gland	193
32	34	39	38	42	40	51	46	26	27	F		

Table 2 Series MB1 no. 19

Table 2 Registrations - *continued*

ICD (9th Revision) number	Site description		All ages	Age-group								
				Under 1	1-4	5-9	10-14	15-19	20-24	25-29	30-34	35-39
194	Malignant neoplasm of other endocrine glands and related structures	M F	65 83	6 4	8 7	2 2	1 1	2 4	4 3	3 2	1 4	3 -
195	Malignant neoplasm of other and ill-defined sites	M F	148 268	4 -	1 1	- -	1 -	1 2	- 1	1 1	2 1	- 1
196	Secondary and unspecified malignant neoplasm of lymph nodes	M F	314 270	- -	- -	- -	- -	- -	1 1	- -	4 3	4 9
197	Secondary malignant neoplasm of respiratory and digestive systems	M F	1,654 1,710	- -	- -	- -	- -	1 -	1 1	1 2	6 8	15 12
198	Secondary malignant neoplasm of other specified sites	M F	808 825	- -	- -	- -	- -	1 1	- -	2 2	6 2	9 7
199	Malignant neoplasm without specification of site	M F	2,316 2,493	- -	- 2	- -	1 -	3 2	2 3	6 3	8 6	16 14
200	Lymphosarcoma and reticulosarcoma	M F	303 231	- -	- -	4 1	4 1	7 2	10 2	5 2	3 2	5 5
201	Hodgkin's disease	M F	693 460	- -	2 1	8 4	25 8	69 50	76 61	87 48	58 57	42 32
202	Other malignant neoplasm of lymphoid and histiocytic tissue	M F	2,174 1,924	3 1	9 2	21 1	9 6	21 12	38 27	30 22	49 26	74 54
203	Multiple myeloma and immunoproliferative neoplasms	M F	1,152 1,018	- -	- -	- -	- -	1 -	- 1	1 1	4 5	5 8
204-208	All leukaemias	M F	2,123 1,801	5 14	81 61	42 35	40 22	61 30	30 21	34 26	31 27	41 36
204	Lymphoid leukaemia	M F	938 710	2 8	72 48	31 27	26 13	38 17	11 8	11 9	10 5	11 8
205	Myeloid leukaemia	M F	978 904	- -	7 9	9 5	13 7	21 13	19 12	21 16	17 21	28 28
206	Monocytic leukaemia	M F	41 51	- 2	1 1	- 1	- -	- -	- 1	1 1	2 -	1 -
207	Other specified leukaemia	M F	22 18	1 2	- 3	- -	1 1	- -	- -	- -	- -	- -
208	Leukaemia of unspecified cell type	M F	144 118	2 2	1 -	2 2	- 1	2 -	- -	1 -	2 1	1 -
223.3	Benign neoplasm of bladder	M F	28 14	- -	- -	- -	- -	- -	- -	3 -	1 -	- 1
225	Benign neoplasm of brain and other parts of nervous system	M F	288 558	- 1	2 4	5 1	2 2	1 3	2 -	7 6	11 17	10 27
227.3	Benign neoplasm of pituitary gland and craniopharyngeal duct	M F	163 152	- -	- -	- -	- -	3 1	6 11	5 10	4 13	11 12
227.4	Benign neoplasm of pineal gland	M F	- 1	- -	- -	- 1	- -	- -	- -	- -	- -	- -
230	Carcinoma in situ of digestive organs	M F	103 81	- -	- -	- -	- -	- -	- -	- -	- -	1 -
231	Carcinoma in situ of respiratory systems	M F	112 48	- -	- -	- 1	- -	- -	- -	- -	- 2	- -
232	Carcinoma in situ of skin	M F	629 1,048	- -	- -	- -	- -	1 -	- 2	1 1	2 6	13 13
233	Carcinoma in situ of breast and genitourinary system	M F	261 14,659	- -	- 1	- -	1 -	- 149	1 1,361	1 3,063	2 3,168	3 2,724

40-44	45-49	50-54	55-59	60-64	65-69	70-74	75-79	80-84	85 and over		Site description	ICD (9th Revision) number
2	4	4	3	7	6	1	6	2	-	M	Malignant neoplasm of other endocrine glands and related structures	194
5	3	4	6	7	10	11	5	1	4	F		
1	4	10	20	17	16	27	22	12	9	M	Malignant neoplasm of other and ill-defined sites	195
2	5	8	13	28	28	42	44	40	51	F		
13	16	20	26	47	42	54	57	20	10	M	Secondary and unspecified malignant neoplasm of lymph nodes	196
6	11	16	30	36	38	42	38	27	13	F		
16	30	79	116	209	283	321	289	195	92	M	Secondary malignant neoplasm of respiratory and digestive systems	197
18	26	68	106	178	232	286	313	258	202	F		
13	20	36	81	135	150	150	106	73	26	M	Secondary malignant neoplasm of other specified sites	198
16	26	40	76	98	118	142	150	89	58	F		
22	28	57	149	264	335	469	412	342	202	M	Malignant neoplasm without specification of site	199
18	35	69	123	207	241	403	464	449	454	F		
10	14	22	26	43	37	46	26	33	8	M	Lymphosarcoma and reticulosarcoma	200
7	9	15	15	28	26	42	30	24	20	F		
59	45	35	39	41	35	31	21	13	7	M	Hodgkin's disease	201
22	13	12	16	18	34	27	27	18	12	F		
84	110	159	229	281	279	305	259	146	68	M	Other malignant neoplasm of lymphoid and histiocytic tissue	202
62	75	125	160	188	247	297	280	212	127	F		
13	38	61	91	140	156	246	201	120	75	M	Multiple myeloma and immunoproliferative neoplasms	203
6	16	47	75	86	132	167	210	158	106	F		
57	47	89	120	204	236	308	348	216	133	M	All leukaemias	204-208
40	44	59	86	134	173	218	250	270	255	F		
14	16	33	48	81	99	131	149	96	59	M	Lymphoid leukaemia	204
6	12	13	28	34	57	76	102	123	116	F		
40	27	50	67	102	107	142	148	98	62	M	Myeloid leukaemia	205
27	27	40	56	89	98	121	112	111	112	F		
-	-	1	1	5	4	9	9	2	5	M	Monocytic leukaemia	206
2	2	3	1	2	4	6	10	12	3	F		
-	1	1	-	1	5	4	6	2	-	M	Other specified leukaemia	207
-	-	1	-	1	1	2	3	-	4	F		
3	3	4	4	15	21	22	36	18	7	M	Leukaemia of unspecified cell type	208
5	3	2	1	8	13	13	23	24	20	F		
1	1	1	-	5	6	5	4	1	-	M	Benign neoplasm of bladder	223.3
1	4	-	3	1	1	1	1	-	-	F		
25	22	20	39	41	36	29	24	8	4	M	Benign neoplasm of brain and other parts of nervous system	225
43	48	37	60	85	72	64	42	30	16	F		
13	16	18	28	24	13	10	7	3	2	M	Benign neoplasm of pituitary gland and craniopharyngeal duct	227.3
11	13	10	20	20	9	14	5	2	1	F		
-	-	-	-	-	-	-	-	-	-	M	Benign neoplasm of pineal gland	227.4
-	-	-	-	-	-	-	-	-	-	F		
3	5	10	12	12	19	23	15	2	1	M	Carcinoma in situ of digestive organs	230
2	4	3	10	5	12	17	12	10	6	F		
3	2	6	10	20	19	33	14	4	1	M	Carcinoma in situ of respiratory systems	231
1	3	5	5	8	11	5	5	2	-	F		
7	21	28	50	78	108	138	92	60	30	M	Carcinoma in situ of skin	232
24	35	38	70	150	140	181	169	137	82	F		
7	13	11	27	33	57	45	36	14	10	M	Carcinoma in situ of breast and genitourinary system	233
1,638	898	525	357	293	198	130	93	41	20	F		

Table 2 Registrations - *continued*

ICD (9th Revision) number	Site description		All ages	Age-group								
				Under 1	1-4	5-9	10-14	15-19	20-24	25-29	30-34	35-39
233.1	Carcinoma in situ of cervix uteri	F	13,609	-	-	-	-	149	1,352	3,047	3,125	2,648
234	Carcinoma in situ of other and unspecified sites	M F	5 9	- -	- -	- -	- -	- -	- -	- -	- 2	- -
235	Neoplasm of uncertain behaviour of digestive and respiratory systems	M F	310 419	- 1	1 -	- -	2 4	8 18	6 17	13 19	9 20	12 14
236	Neoplasm of uncertain behaviour of genitourinary organs	M F	263 819	- 1	1 -	- -	- 1	3 26	4 98	4 123	4 111	6 97
237	Neoplasm of uncertain behaviour of endocrine glands and nervous system	M F	157 165	2 -	1 3	7 3	7 10	15 11	8 8	7 12	3 8	6 9
238	Neoplasm of uncertain behaviour of other and unspecified sites and tissues	M F	546 525	1 4	2 4	3 3	1 3	4 4	15 9	7 9	5 11	13 15
239.4	Neoplasm of unspecified nature of bladder	M F	48 8	- -	- -	- -	- -	- -	1 -	1 -	1 -	- -
239.6	Neoplasm of unspecified nature of brain	M F	164 174	1 1	3 1	1 -	1 1	1 2	1 2	3 2	2 3	5 6
239.7	Neoplasm of unspecified nature of other parts of nervous system and pituitary gland only	M F	33 26	1 -	- -	2 1	- -	1 1	- 2	2 1	- 1	2 2
630	Hydatidiform mole	F	171	-	-	-	-	26	46	54	33	7

40-44	45-49	50-54	55-59	60-64	65-69	70-74	75-79	80-84	85 and over		Site description	ICD (9th Revision) number
1,520	759	383	251	195	96	48	21	8	7	F	Carcinoma in situ of cervix uteri	233.1
-	-	-	-	2	2	1	-	-	-	M	Carcinoma in situ of other and	234
1	-	1	-	2	1	-	1	-	1	F	unspecified sites	
10	9	22	30	30	40	48	46	18	6	M	Neoplasm of uncertain behaviour of	235
15	17	20	32	35	48	62	48	32	17	F	digestive and respiratory systems	
6	14	18	26	43	29	42	28	21	14	M	Neoplasm of uncertain behaviour of	236
67	35	44	31	52	38	35	32	16	12	F	genitourinary organs	
10	10	13	13	15	17	9	9	3	2	M	Neoplasm of uncertain behaviour of	237
16	9	14	8	11	9	12	10	6	6	F	endocrine glands and nervous system	
16	20	24	51	63	71	95	77	56	22	M	Neoplasm of uncertain behaviour of	238
14	25	23	35	48	45	87	81	51	54	F	other and unspecified sites and tissues	
1	-	2	2	7	7	7	8	8	3	M	Neoplasm of unspecified nature of	239.4
-	-	1	1	1	-	-	2	2	1	F	bladder	
6	9	10	17	18	24	24	20	12	6	M	Neoplasm of unspecified nature of	239.6
4	3	8	7	11	22	27	35	16	23	F	brain	
1	2	-	3	7	6	3	1	-	2	M	Neoplasm of unspecified nature of	239.7
1	-	-	3	3	3	2	4	2	-	F	other parts of nervous system and pituitary gland only	
-	4	1	-	-	-	-	-	-	-	F	Hydatidiform mole	630

Series MB1 no. 19 Table 2

21

Table 3 Series MB1 no. 19

Table 3 Rates per 100,000 population of newly diagnosed cases of cancer : sex, site and age, 1986

ICD (9th Revision) number	Site description		All ages	Under 1	1-4	5-9	10-14	15-19	20-24	25-29	30-34	35-39
	All registrations	M	436.8	14.6	15.0	9.7	10.2	18.4	23.0	35.6	44.3	68.5
		F	472.1	17.6	12.4	7.6	8.6	24.8	94.6	219.9	287.8	297.8
140-208	All malignant neoplasms	M	424.1	13.1	14.3	8.5	9.3	16.6	21.0	32.8	41.7	64.1
		F	398.5	15.1	11.4	6.9	7.2	12.2	19.5	41.2	83.1	139.4
140	Malignant neoplasm of lip	M	0.8	-	-	-	-	0.0	-	0.1	-	0.2
		F	0.2	-	-	-	-	-	-	-	-	0.1
141	Malignant neoplasm of tongue	M	1.3	-	-	-	-	0.0	0.0	0.1	0.3	0.2
		F	0.8	-	-	-	-	-	0.1	-	0.1	0.4
142	Malignant neoplasm of major salivary glands	M	0.7	-	-	-	0.1	0.0	0.1	0.1	0.2	0.3
		F	0.6	-	-	-	0.1	-	0.0	0.1	0.3	0.2
143	Malignant neoplasm of gum	M	0.3	-	-	-	-	-	-	-	-	0.1
		F	0.2	-	-	-	-	-	-	-	-	0.1
144	Malignant neoplasm of floor of mouth	M	0.9	-	-	-	-	-	-	-	-	0.2
		F	0.2	-	-	-	-	-	-	-	-	-
145	Malignant neoplasm of other and unspecified parts of mouth	M	0.8	-	-	-	0.1	0.0	-	0.1	0.1	0.1
		F	0.5	-	-	-	-	-	-	0.1	0.1	0.1
146	Malignant neoplasm of oropharynx	M	0.9	-	-	0.1	-	-	-	-	-	0.2
		F	0.4	-	-	-	-	-	0.0	-	0.2	0.1
147	Malignant neoplasm of nasopharynx	M	0.4	-	-	0.1	0.1	0.1	0.0	0.1	0.1	0.2
		F	0.2	-	-	0.1	-	0.2	0.1	0.2	-	0.3
148	Malignant neoplasm of hypopharynx	M	0.8	-	-	-	-	-	0.0	-	-	-
		F	0.5	-	-	-	-	-	-	-	-	0.1
149	Malignant neoplasm of other and ill-defined sites within the lip, oral cavity and pharynx	M	0.4	-	-	-	-	-	0.0	-	-	0.1
		F	0.2	-	-	-	-	-	-	-	-	0.2
150	Malignant neoplasm of oesophagus	M	10.6	-	-	-	-	-	0.0	0.1	0.4	1.1
		F	7.1	-	-	-	-	-	-	-	0.1	0.3
151	Malignant neoplasm of stomach	M	27.1	-	-	-	-	0.0	0.0	0.5	0.5	2.1
		F	15.7	-	-	-	-	-	0.1	0.3	0.5	1.0
152	Malignant neoplasm of small intestine, including duodenum	M	0.6	-	0.1	-	-	0.0	-	0.1	0.1	0.2
		F	0.6	-	-	-	-	-	-	-	0.2	0.1
153	Malignant neoplasm of colon	M	26.8	-	-	-	-	0.1	0.2	0.6	1.2	3.3
		F	32.1	-	-	-	-	0.1	0.2	0.5	1.4	3.4
154	Malignant neoplasm of rectum, rectosigmoid junction and anus	M	21.2	-	-	0.1	-	0.0	0.2	0.5	0.8	1.9
		F	16.2	0.3	-	-	-	-	0.0	0.2	0.7	1.4
155	Malignant neoplasm of liver and intrahepatic bile ducts	M	2.5	0.3	0.2	0.1	0.1	0.0	-	0.3	0.4	0.5
		F	1.5	0.3	0.1	0.2	0.1	-	0.2	-	0.3	0.3
156	Malignant neoplasm of gallbladder and extrahepatic bile ducts	M	2.0	-	-	-	-	0.0	-	0.1	-	0.1
		F	2.7	-	-	-	-	-	-	-	0.1	0.3
157	Malignant neoplasm of pancreas	M	11.3	0.3	-	-	0.1	-	-	0.3	0.4	0.8
		F	11.0	-	-	-	0.1	0.1	-	0.1	0.2	0.8
158	Malignant neoplasm of retroperitoneum and peritoneum	M	0.4	-	-	-	-	0.0	0.2	0.1	0.1	0.1
		F	0.5	-	0.1	-	-	0.1	0.0	0.1	0.2	0.1
159	Malignant neoplasm of other and ill-defined sites within the digestive organs and peritoneum	M	0.7	-	-	-	-	-	0.0	-	-	0.1
		F	0.8	-	-	-	-	-	0.0	0.1	-	0.1
160	Malignant neoplasm of nasal cavities, middle ear and accessory sinuses	M	0.9	-	-	0.1	0.1	0.1	0.0	0.1	-	0.3
		F	0.6	-	-	-	0.1	-	0.0	0.1	-	0.3
161	Malignant neoplasm of larynx	M	6.0	-	-	-	-	-	-	0.1	0.1	0.4
		F	1.2	-	-	-	-	0.1	-	0.1	0.2	0.1

England and Wales

40-44	45-49	50-54	55-59	60-64	65-69	70-74	75-79	80-84	85 and over		Site description	ICD (9th Revision) number
112.7	**198.1**	**356.6**	**636.6**	**1079.5**	**1571.8**	**2202.8**	**2846.8**	**3317.8**	**3642.7**	M	**All registrations**	
331.1	**396.4**	**497.9**	**643.4**	**858.7**	**1039.9**	**1285.6**	**1494.2**	**1706.8**	**2022.0**	F		
105.8	**187.8**	**342.9**	**613.4**	**1048.9**	**1529.5**	**2145.8**	**2786.0**	**3253.3**	**3574.0**	M	**All malignant neoplasms**	140-2
214.0	**316.9**	**443.1**	**596.7**	**807.5**	**992.3**	**1232.9**	**1441.0**	**1656.5**	**1973.1**	F		
0.3	0.6	0.7	0.8	2.0	3.8	2.9	6.1	5.2	7.3	M	Malignant neoplasm of lip	140
0.1	-	-	0.1	0.1	0.5	1.0	0.7	1.7	1.2	F		
0.9	1.7	2.3	3.0	3.9	4.5	4.0	7.2	5.5	6.0	M	Malignant neoplasm of tongue	141
0.4	0.5	0.9	1.1	1.3	2.0	2.6	3.2	4.5	4.7	F		
0.3	0.6	0.8	0.8	0.7	2.1	3.0	3.2	5.5	6.7	M	Malignant neoplasm of major salivary glands	142
0.8	0.6	0.7	0.7	0.7	1.3	1.8	1.7	2.9	3.3	F		
0.1	0.1	0.7	0.7	0.6	1.1	1.1	2.4	0.9	2.0	M	Malignant neoplasm of gum	143
0.1	0.1	0.2	0.1	0.6	0.4	0.7	0.2	1.0	1.4	F		
0.3	1.5	1.6	2.6	3.3	3.2	2.9	2.6	1.5	4.0	M	Malignant neoplasm of floor of mouth	144
-	0.1	0.3	0.4	1.0	0.5	0.6	0.7	1.2	1.0	F		
0.4	0.7	1.0	2.0	2.7	2.9	2.8	3.2	4.6	6.7	M	Malignant neoplasm of other and unspecified parts of mouth	145
0.1	0.5	1.1	0.7	1.1	1.9	1.7	2.3	1.9	1.4	F		
0.7	1.0	1.4	2.2	2.7	3.2	2.7	3.7	3.7	4.7	M	Malignant neoplasm of oropharynx	146
0.3	0.3	0.5	0.7	1.3	1.3	1.1	0.8	1.2	1.2	F		
0.3	0.9	0.7	0.8	1.4	1.4	1.2	1.1	2.5	0.7	M	Malignant neoplasm of nasopharynx	147
0.1	0.1	0.5	0.3	0.6	0.5	0.4	0.6	0.6	0.4	F		
0.2	0.8	1.3	2.0	3.5	2.5	4.0	3.5	3.4	4.7	M	Malignant neoplasm of hypopharynx	148
0.1	0.3	0.8	0.8	0.8	2.1	2.1	2.0	1.9	1.8	F		
0.1	0.4	0.4	0.8	1.4	1.5	1.6	1.4	1.5	2.7	M	Malignant neoplasm of other and ill-defined sites within the lip, oral cavity and pharynx	149
-	0.1	0.4	0.2	0.4	0.3	0.7	0.7	0.3	0.8	F		
1.8	5.2	9.3	18.0	28.2	40.2	53.9	67.3	79.8	88.7	M	Malignant neoplasm of oesophagus	150
0.9	2.1	3.2	8.7	11.5	17.5	24.7	34.8	42.7	54.6	F		
3.6	9.3	18.3	38.5	64.2	99.9	144.3	201.5	238.4	256.7	M	Malignant neoplasm of stomach	151
2.0	3.8	7.1	10.6	22.3	32.6	53.0	82.7	111.4	141.3	F		
0.2	0.7	1.0	1.4	1.8	1.9	2.1	3.0	3.7	4.7	M	Malignant neoplasm of small intestine, including duodenum	152
0.1	0.2	0.8	1.0	1.9	1.0	2.2	2.7	3.0	2.2	F		
5.8	10.8	20.8	39.1	61.1	91.6	134.9	192.4	241.8	284.1	M	Malignant neoplasm of colon	153
6.9	12.2	24.8	37.5	58.1	73.0	103.5	147.6	188.9	246.6	F		
5.3	9.2	19.3	32.4	56.3	77.1	108.2	144.4	159.9	166.0	M	Malignant neoplasm of rectum, rectosigmoid junction and anus	154
3.5	7.2	12.3	20.8	30.4	40.1	56.2	70.3	84.5	121.5	F		
0.9	1.3	3.0	3.6	6.4	10.0	12.3	13.7	13.5	14.0	M	Malignant neoplasm of liver and intrahepatic bile ducts	155
0.2	0.5	0.8	2.0	3.0	3.5	5.0	6.5	7.3	11.7	F		
0.3	1.1	1.6	2.6	4.8	7.7	9.6	13.6	15.3	20.7	M	Malignant neoplasm of gallbladder and extrahepatic bile ducts	156
0.6	0.9	1.6	3.6	3.6	5.7	10.3	13.7	16.6	19.0	F		
2.2	4.4	9.2	16.6	29.9	43.9	58.2	76.5	83.2	105.4	M	Malignant neoplasm of pancreas	157
1.1	2.6	6.2	9.9	17.9	28.8	40.8	57.1	64.3	81.6	F		
0.3	0.4	0.4	0.6	1.9	1.7	1.2	1.9	1.2	1.3	M	Malignant neoplasm of retroperitoneum and peritoneum	158
0.2	0.7	0.5	0.5	1.3	1.2	1.4	1.8	1.7	1.0	F		
0.2	0.1	0.4	1.0	1.5	3.3	2.7	5.0	7.1	7.3	M	Malignant neoplasm of other and ill-defined sites within the digestive organs and peritoneum	159
-	0.1	0.5	0.4	1.1	1.0	2.6	3.3	5.4	10.0	F		
0.3	0.6	1.0	1.7	2.3	2.7	4.5	4.5	4.3	6.0	M	Malignant neoplasm of nasal cavities, middle ear and accessory sinuses	160
0.1	0.5	0.8	0.7	1.3	1.4	1.4	2.3	3.2	4.1	F		
1.9	3.5	7.6	13.4	21.7	24.5	29.4	24.4	27.0	30.0	M	Malignant neoplasm of larynx	161
0.6	1.0	1.4	2.2	4.8	4.1	4.0	3.5	2.3	4.3	F		

Table 3 Series MB1 no. 19

Table 3 Rates per 100,000 population - *continued*

ICD (9th Revision) number	Site description		All ages	Under 1	1-4	5-9	10-14	15-19	20-24	25-29	30-34	35-39
162	Malignant neoplasm of trachea, bronchus and lung	M F	**99.8** **38.9**	- -	- -	0.1 -	- 0.1	0.0 0.1	0.2 0.0	0.4 0.6	1.6 0.8	4.4 3.2
163	Malignant neoplasm of pleura	M F	**2.1** **0.4**	- -	- -	- -	- -	- -	- -	- -	0.1 -	0.4 0.2
164	Malignant neoplasm of thymus, heart and mediastinum	M F	**0.3** **0.2**	- 0.3	0.1 -	- 0.1	0.1 -	0.1 -	0.2 -	0.2 0.1	0.3 0.1	0.2 0.2
165	Malignant neoplasm of other and ill-defined sites within the respiratory system and intrathoracic organs	M F	**0.0** **0.0**	- -	- -	- -	- -	- -	- -	- -	- -	- -
170	Malignant neoplasm of bone and articular cartilage	M F	**0.9** **0.8**	0.6 0.6	0.1 0.3	0.4 0.4	0.7 1.1	1.6 0.9	0.9 1.0	0.3 0.3	0.2 0.4	0.5 0.5
171	Malignant neoplasm of connective and other soft tissue	M F	**1.9** **1.6**	0.3 1.9	0.5 0.7	0.5 0.2	0.5 0.6	0.8 0.7	0.8 0.5	0.7 0.6	0.8 0.7	1.4 1.2
172	Malignant melanoma of skin	M F	**4.1** **7.1**	- -	0.1 -	0.1 0.1	0.2 0.3	0.4 1.0	1.2 2.1	2.6 4.5	2.5 5.8	3.8 7.2
173	Other malignant neoplasm of skin	M F	**58.0** **49.1**	- 0.6	- 0.2	- 0.1	0.3 0.3	0.4 0.5	0.5 1.2	2.1 1.9	5.1 6.3	9.9 11.3
174	Malignant neoplasm of female breast	F	**88.6**	0.3	-	-	0.1	0.2	0.9	6.6	22.8	53.2
175	Malignant neoplasm of male breast	M	**0.6**	-	-	-	-	-	-	0.1	0.1	0.2
179	Malignant neoplasm of uterus, part unspecified	F	**1.5**	-	-	-	-	-	-	-	0.4	0.4
180	Malignant neoplasm of cervix uteri	F	**15.7**	-	-	-	0.1	-	2.0	12.3	22.4	26.3
181	Malignant neoplasm of placenta	F	**0.0**	-	-	-	-	0.1	0.0	0.2	0.2	0.1
182	Malignant neoplasm of body of uterus	F	**13.4**	-	-	-	-	0.1	0.0	0.3	0.8	1.9
183	Malignant neoplasm of ovary and other uterine adnexa	F	**17.6**	-	0.2	-	0.3	0.8	1.5	1.9	3.7	6.2
184	Malignant neoplasm of other and unspecified female genital organs	F	**3.8**	-	-	-	-	-	0.1	0.5	0.9	0.8
185	Malignant neoplasm of prostate	M	**41.7**	-	-	-	-	-	0.0	0.1	-	0.1
186	Malignant neoplasm of testis	M	**4.2**	1.2	0.7	-	-	2.2	5.8	10.3	10.2	8.7
187	Malignant neoplasm of penis and other male genital organs	M	**1.3**	-	-	-	-	0.0	0.0	0.1	0.2	0.4
188	Malignant neoplasm of bladder	M F	**27.8** **10.9**	- 0.3	- -	0.1 -	0.1 -	0.0 0.1	0.6 0.1	0.6 0.2	1.8 0.3	2.4 0.9
189	Malignant neoplasm of kidney and other and unspecified urinary organs	M F	**7.8** **4.6**	0.9 0.6	1.2 1.5	0.4 0.7	- -	0.0 -	0.2 0.1	0.5 0.3	0.5 0.5	2.0 1.1
190	Malignant neoplasm of eye	M F	**0.8** **0.6**	3.0 1.9	0.5 0.5	0.1 -	- -	0.0 -	0.1 0.1	0.1 -	0.2 0.3	0.3 0.3
191	Malignant neoplasm of brain	M F	**6.2** **4.3**	0.9 1.3	2.7 1.4	1.5 2.1	1.9 1.2	1.0 1.4	1.5 1.4	2.1 1.2	2.4 1.7	5.0 3.0
192	Malignant neoplasm of other and unspecified parts of nervous system	M F	**0.2** **0.2**	0.3 0.6	0.4 0.4	0.2 0.1	0.2 0.3	0.1 0.1	0.0 -	0.3 -	0.1 0.2	0.2 0.2
193	Malignant neoplasm of thyroid gland	M F	**0.9** **2.0**	- -	- -	- -	0.1 0.2	0.3 0.5	0.1 1.4	0.3 1.8	0.8 1.7	0.4 2.3

40-44	45-49	50-54	55-59	60-64	65-69	70-74	75-79	80-84	85 and over		Site description	ICD (9th Revision) number
11.6	32.6	64.9	152.3	282.6	415.2	559.8	670.2	720.1	684.8	M	Malignant neoplasm of trachea, bronchus and lung	162
6.3	15.1	29.3	61.9	107.9	141.2	159.7	147.7	143.6	122.9	F		
1.3	1.1	3.1	4.9	7.5	8.8	8.2	7.8	10.1	4.7	M	Malignant neoplasm of pleura	163
0.3	0.1	0.2	0.7	1.3	1.3	1.1	1.2	1.6	0.8	F		
0.1	0.1	0.3	0.8	0.8	0.2	1.1	0.8	0.9	-	M	Malignant neoplasm of thymus, heart and mediastinum	164
0.2	0.1	0.5	0.4	0.1	0.6	0.4	0.6	0.3	0.6	F		
-	-	0.1	-	0.1	-	0.2	0.2	-	0.7	M	Malignant neoplasm of other and ill-defined sites within the respiratory system and intrathoracic organs	165
-	-	-	-	-	0.1	-	-	-	-	F		
0.7	0.6	1.0	1.4	1.8	1.9	2.0	1.8	1.8	2.7	M	Malignant neoplasm of bone and articular cartilage	170
0.5	0.4	0.8	0.9	0.8	1.3	1.7	1.7	2.0	2.5	F		
1.9	1.1	2.3	2.9	4.0	4.1	5.6	7.7	8.3	6.7	M	Malignant neoplasm of connective and other soft tissue	171
1.0	1.3	2.6	2.5	2.3	2.8	3.6	4.4	4.2	7.8	F		
4.8	5.6	7.5	6.4	9.9	10.2	8.5	12.0	11.7	15.3	M	Malignant melanoma of skin	172
10.6	9.8	11.6	11.1	12.7	15.2	13.6	13.2	12.5	13.1	F		
17.8	30.8	58.4	90.5	149.3	208.2	282.9	364.1	421.3	510.8	M	Other malignant neoplasm of skin	173
18.2	28.9	38.6	57.3	86.3	119.7	166.2	212.1	262.0	310.8	F		
94.3	136.8	154.4	167.7	197.9	204.6	221.3	229.4	240.9	293.4	F	Malignant neoplasm of female breast	174
0.3	0.6	0.8	1.0	1.5	1.7	2.9	3.7	3.7	8.0	M	Malignant neoplasm of male breast	175
0.4	0.9	2.3	2.5	3.5	3.8	4.3	5.3	4.2	10.2	F	Malignant neoplasm of uterus, part unspecified	179
23.3	24.4	20.9	23.2	30.7	30.2	25.6	22.9	18.4	23.5	F	Malignant neoplasm of cervix uteri	180
0.1	-	-	-	-	-	-	-	-	-	F	Malignant neoplasm of placenta	181
4.2	10.7	24.6	37.6	35.0	37.6	40.7	39.3	39.1	37.0	F	Malignant neoplasm of body of uterus	182
13.1	19.4	30.8	40.5	39.5	47.1	50.2	48.6	46.8	44.2	F	Malignant neoplasm of ovary and other uterine adnexa	183
0.8	1.0	3.0	3.3	5.2	7.3	13.6	17.8	23.4	30.5	F	Malignant neoplasm of other and unspecified female genital organs	184
0.7	1.6	7.2	25.9	64.6	139.2	259.4	386.2	530.5	599.4	M	Malignant neoplasm of prostate	185
7.7	4.2	3.4	2.0	1.7	1.0	1.6	1.6	1.5	1.3	M	Malignant neoplasm of testis	186
0.6	0.9	1.2	1.8	2.2	3.8	5.9	10.5	9.2	14.7	M	Malignant neoplasm of penis and other male genital organs	187
4.8	11.4	21.7	40.6	71.3	101.8	148.7	195.2	212.9	231.4	M	Malignant neoplasm of bladder	188
1.5	3.7	8.6	13.4	21.9	29.6	42.1	47.6	57.5	67.3	F		
2.8	5.8	12.6	15.3	21.8	29.1	32.8	43.5	37.1	30.0	M	Malignant neoplasm of kidney and other and unspecified urinary organs	189
2.0	3.5	4.9	6.8	10.5	12.7	16.8	16.6	17.1	16.8	F		
0.4	0.9	1.0	1.3	1.7	2.5	2.2	3.8	2.1	1.3	M	Malignant neoplasm of eye	190
0.3	0.4	0.8	1.3	1.5	0.9	1.3	2.5	1.5	1.6	F		
5.4	9.0	9.9	12.2	16.8	21.4	15.5	11.7	8.6	8.0	M	Malignant neoplasm of brain	191
3.8	4.7	5.9	8.2	11.0	12.3	9.6	8.0	4.5	3.1	F		
-	0.3	0.2	0.2	0.5	0.3	0.4	0.5-	-	-	M	Malignant neoplasm of other and unspecified parts of nervous system	192
0.3	0.1	0.5	0.4	0.1	0.5	0.3	-	0.1	-	F		
0.6	0.7	1.2	2.1	1.8	2.6	2.3	3.2	4.3	4.0	M	Malignant neoplasm of thyroid gland	193
2.0	2.5	2.9	2.8	3.0	3.1	4.2	4.5	5.5	3.8	F		

Table 3 Series MB1 no. 19

Table 3 Rates per 100,000 population - *continued*

ICD (9th Revision) number	Site description		All ages	Under 1	1-4	5-9	10-14	15-19	20-24	25-29	30-34	35-39
194	Malignant neoplasm of other endocrine glands and related structures	M	0.3	1.8	0.6	0.1	0.1	0.1	0.2	0.2	0.1	0.2
		F	0.3	1.3	0.6	0.1	0.1	0.2	0.1	0.1	0.2	-
195	Malignant neoplasm of other and ill-defined sites	M	0.6	1.2	0.1	-	0.1	0.0	-	0.1	0.1	-
		F	1.0	-	0.1	-	-	0.1	0.0	0.1	0.1	0.1
196	Secondary and unspecified malignant neoplasm of lymph nodes	M	1.3	-	-	-	-	-	0.0	-	0.2	0.2
		F	1.1	-	-	-	-	-	0.0	-	0.2	0.5
197	Secondary malignant neoplasm of respiratory and digestive systems	M	6.8	-	-	-	-	0.0	0.0	0.1	0.4	0.8
		F	6.7	-	-	-	-	-	0.0	0.1	0.5	0.6
198	Secondary malignant neoplasm of other specified sites	M	3.3	-	-	-	-	0.0	-	0.1	0.4	0.5
		F	3.2	-	-	-	-	0.1	-	0.1	0.1	0.4
199	Malignant neoplasm without specification of site	M	9.5	-	-	-	0.1	0.1	0.1	0.3	0.5	0.9
		F	9.7	-	0.2	-	-	0.1	0.1	0.2	0.4	0.8
200	Lymphosarcoma and reticulosarcoma	M	1.2	-	-	0.3	0.2	0.3	0.5	0.3	0.2	0.3
		F	0.9	-	-	0.1	0.1	0.1	0.1	0.1	0.1	0.3
201	Hodgkin's disease	M	2.8	-	0.2	0.5	1.5	3.4	3.6	4.6	3.4	2.3
		F	1.8	-	0.1	0.3	0.5	2.6	2.9	2.6	3.4	1.7
202	Other malignant neoplasm of lymphoid and histiocytic tissue	M	8.9	0.9	0.7	1.4	0.5	1.0	1.8	1.6	2.9	4.0
		F	7.5	0.3	0.2	0.1	0.4	0.6	1.3	1.2	1.6	2.9
203	Multiple myeloma and immunoproliferative neoplasms	M	4.7	-	-	-	-	0.0	-	0.1	0.2	0.3
		F	4.0	-	-	-	-	-	0.0	0.1	0.3	0.4
204-208	All leukaemias	M	8.7	1.5	6.2	2.7	2.4	3.0	1.4	1.8	1.8	2.2
		F	7.0	4.4	5.0	2.4	1.4	1.6	1.0	1.4	1.6	1.9
204	Lymphoid leukaemia	M	3.8	0.6	5.6	2.0	1.6	1.9	0.5	0.6	0.6	0.6
		F	2.8	2.5	3.9	1.8	0.8	0.9	0.4	0.5	0.3	0.4
205	Myeloid leukaemia	M	4.0	-	0.5	0.6	0.8	1.0	0.9	1.1	1.0	1.5
		F	3.5	-	0.7	0.3	0.4	0.7	0.6	0.9	1.3	1.5
206	Monocytic leukaemia	M	0.2	-	0.1	-	-	-	-	0.1	0.1	0.1
		F	0.2	0.6	0.1	0.1	-	-	0.0	0.1	-	-
207	Other specified leukaemia	M	0.1	0.3	-	-	0.1	-	-	-	-	-
		F	0.1	0.6	0.2	-	0.1	-	-	-	-	-
208	Leukaemia of unspecified cell type	M	0.6	0.6	0.1	0.1	-	0.1	-	0.1	0.1	0.1
		F	0.5	0.6	-	0.1	0.1	-	-	-	0.1	-
223.3	Benign neoplasm of bladder	M	0.1	-	-	-	-	-	-	0.2	0.1	-
		F	0.1	-	-	-	-	-	-	0.1	-	0.1
225	Benign neoplasm of brain and other parts of nervous system	M	1.2	-	0.2	0.3	0.1	0.0	0.1	0.4	0.7	0.5
		F	2.2	0.3	0.3	0.1	0.1	0.2	-	0.3	1.0	1.5
227.3	Benign neoplasm of pituitary gland and craniopharyngeal duct	M	0.7	-	-	-	-	0.1	0.3	0.3	0.2	0.6
		F	0.6	-	-	-	-	0.1	0.5	0.5	0.8	0.6
227.4	Benign neoplasm of pineal gland	M	-	-	-	-	-	-	-	-	-	-
		F	0.0	-	-	0.1	-	-	-	-	-	-
230	Carcinoma in situ of digestive organs	M	0.4	-	-	-	-	-	-	-	-	0.1
		F	0.3	-	-	-	-	-	-	-	-	-
231	Carcinoma in situ of respiratory systems	M	0.5	-	-	-	-	-	-	-	-	-
		F	0.2	-	-	0.1	-	-	-	-	0.1	-
232	Carcinoma in situ of skin	M	2.6	-	-	-	-	0.0	-	0.1	0.1	0.7
		F	4.1	-	-	-	-	-	0.1	0.1	0.4	0.7
233	Carcinoma in situ of breast and genitourinary system	M	1.1	-	-	-	0.1	-	0.0	0.1	0.1	0.2
		F	57.1	-	0.1	-	-	7.8	65.7	165.8	191.0	147.3

Series MB1 no. 19 Table 3

40-44	45-49	50-54	55-59	60-64	65-69	70-74	75-79	80-84	85 and over		Site description	ICD (9th Revision) number
0.1	*0.3*	*0.3*	*0.2*	*0.5*	*0.6*	*0.1*	*1.0*	*0.6*	-	M	Malignant neoplasm of other endocrine glands and related structures	194
0.3	*0.2*	*0.3*	*0.4*	*0.5*	*0.8*	*0.9*	*0.5*	*0.1*	*0.8*	F		
0.1	*0.3*	*0.7*	1.5	*1.3*	*1.5*	3.0	3.5	*3.7*	6.0	M	Malignant neoplasm of other and ill-defined sites	195
0.1	*0.4*	*0.6*	0.9	2.0	2.2	3.5	4.3	5.8	10.4	F		
0.8	*1.1*	1.5	2.0	3.6	3.9	6.0	9.1	6.1	6.7	M	Secondary and unspecified malignant neoplasm of lymph nodes	196
0.4	0.8	*1.2*	2.2	2.5	3.0	3.5	3.7	3.9	2.7	F		
1.0	2.2	5.9	8.7	16.1	26.4	35.8	46.2	59.8	61.3	M	Secondary malignant neoplasm of respiratory and digestive systems	197
1.1	1.9	5.1	7.7	12.6	18.1	23.6	30.9	37.5	41.3	F		
0.8	1.4	2.7	6.1	10.4	14.0	16.7	16.9	22.4	17.3	M	Secondary malignant neoplasm of other specified sites	198
1.0	1.9	3.0	5.5	6.9	9.2	11.7	14.8	12.9	11.9	F		
1.4	2.0	4.3	11.2	20.3	31.3	52.3	65.8	104.9	134.7	M	Malignant neoplasm without specification of site	199
1.1	2.5	5.2	9.0	14.6	18.8	33.3	45.8	65.2	92.8	F		
0.6	*1.0*	1.6	2.0	3.3	3.5	5.1	4.2	10.1	*5.3*	M	Lymphosarcoma and reticulosarcoma	200
0.4	0.7	*1.1*	*1.1*	2.0	2.0	3.5	3.0	3.5	4.1	F		
3.7	3.2	2.6	2.9	3.2	3.3	3.5	3.4	*4.0*	*4.7*	M	Hodgkin's disease	201
1.4	0.9	0.9	*1.2*	*1.3*	2.7	2.2	2.7	2.6	*2.5*	F		
5.3	7.9	11.9	17.2	21.6	26.0	34.0	41.4	44.8	45.3	M	Other malignant neoplasm of lymphoid and histiocytic tissue	202
3.9	5.4	9.4	11.6	13.3	19.3	24.5	27.6	30.8	26.0	F		
0.8	2.7	4.6	6.8	10.8	14.6	27.4	32.1	36.8	50.0	M	Multiple myeloma and immunoproliferative neoplasms	203
0.4	*1.2*	3.5	5.5	6.1	10.3	13.8	20.7	22.9	21.7	F		
3.6	3.4	6.7	9.0	15.7	22.0	34.3	55.6	66.3	88.7	M	All leukaemias	204-208
2.5	3.2	4.4	6.3	9.5	13.5	18.0	24.7	39.2	52.1	F		
0.9	*1.1*	2.5	3.6	6.2	9.2	14.6	23.8	29.5	39.3	M	Lymphoid leukaemia	204
0.4	0.9	*1.0*	2.0	2.4	4.5	6.3	10.1	17.9	23.7	F		
2.5	1.9	3.7	5.0	7.8	10.0	15.8	23.6	30.1	41.3	M	Myeloid leukaemia	205
1.7	2.0	3.0	4.1	6.3	7.7	10.0	11.0	16.1	22.9	F		
-	-	*0.1*	*0.1*	0.4	0.4	*1.0*	1.4	0.6	3.3	M	Monocytic leukaemia	206
0.1	*0.1*	0.2	*0.1*	*0.1*	0.3	0.5	*1.0*	1.7	0.6	F		
-	*0.1*	*0.1*	-	*0.1*	0.5	0.4	*1.0*	0.6	-	M	Other specified leukaemia	207
-	-	*0.1*	-	*0.1*	*0.1*	0.2	0.3	-	0.8	F		
0.2	0.2	0.3	0.3	*1.2*	2.0	2.5	5.8	*5.5*	*4.7*	M	Leukaemia of unspecified cell type	208
0.3	0.2	0.2	*0.1*	0.6	*1.0*	*1.1*	2.3	3.5	4.1	F		
0.1	*0.1*	*0.1*	-	0.4	0.6	0.6	0.6	*0.3*	-	M	223.3Benign neoplasm of bladder	
0.1	0.3	-	0.2	*0.1*	*0.1*	*0.1*	*0.1*	-	-	F		
1.6	1.6	1.5	2.9	3.2	3.4	3.2	3.8	*2.5*	2.7	M	Benign neoplasm of brain and other parts of nervous system	225
2.7	3.5	2.8	4.4	6.0	5.6	5.3	4.1	4.4	*3.3*	F		
0.8	*1.1*	*1.3*	2.1	1.8	*1.2*	*1.1*	*1.1*	*0.9*	*1.3*	M	Benign neoplasm of pituitary gland and craniopharyngeal duct	227.3
0.7	0.9	0.8	1.5	1.4	0.7	*1.2*	0.5	0.3	0.2	F		
-	-	-	-	-	-	-	-	-	-	M	Benign neoplasm of pineal gland	227.4
-	-	-	-	-	-	-	-	-	-	F		
0.2	0.4	0.7	0.9	0.9	1.8	2.6	*2.4*	0.6	0.7	M	Carcinoma in situ of digestive organs	230
0.1	0.3	0.2	0.7	0.4	0.9	1.4	*1.2*	*1.5*	*1.2*	F		
0.2	0.1	0.4	0.8	1.5	1.8	3.7	2.2	*1.2*	0.7	M	Carcinoma in situ of respiratory systems	231
0.1	0.2	0.4	0.4	0.6	0.9	0.4	0.5	0.3	-	F		
0.4	1.5	2.1	3.8	6.0	10.1	15.4	14.7	18.4	20.0	M	Carcinoma in situ of skin	232
1.5	2.5	2.9	5.1	10.6	10.9	15.0	16.7	19.9	16.8	F		
0.4	*0.9*	*0.8*	2.0	2.5	5.3	5.0	5.8	*4.3*	6.7	M	Carcinoma in situ of breast and genitourinary system	233
104.3	65.0	39.4	26.0	20.7	15.5	10.7	9.2	6.0	4.1	F		

Table 3 Series MB1 no. 19

Table 3 Rates per 100,000 population - *continued*

ICD (9th Revision) number	Site description		All ages	Under 1	1-4	5-9	10-14	15-19	20-24	25-29	30-34	35-39
233.1	Carcinoma in situ of cervix uteri	F	**53.0**	-	-	-	-	7.8	65.2	165.0	188.4	143.2
234	Carcinoma in situ of other and unspecified sites	M	**0.0**	-	-	-	-	-	-	-	-	-
		F	**0.0**	-	-	-	-	-	-	-	0.1	-
235	Neoplasm of uncertain behaviour of digestive and respiratory systems	M	**1.3**	-	0.1	-	0.1	0.4	0.3	0.7	0.5	0.6
		F	**1.6**	0.3	-	-	0.3	0.9	0.8	1.0	1.2	0.8
236	Neoplasm of uncertain behaviour of genitourinary organs	M	**1.1**	-	0.1	-	-	0.1	0.2	0.2	0.2	0.3
		F	**3.2**	0.3	-	-	0.1	1.4	4.7	6.7	6.7	5.2
237	Neoplasm of uncertain behaviour of endocrine glands and nervous system	M	**0.6**	0.6	0.1	0.5	0.4	0.7	0.4	0.4	0.2	0.3
		F	**0.6**	-	0.2	0.2	0.6	0.6	0.4	0.6	0.5	0.5
238	Neoplasm of uncertain behaviour of other and unspecified sites and tissues	M	**2.2**	0.3	0.2	0.2	0.1	0.2	0.7	0.4	0.3	0.7
		F	**2.0**	1.3	0.3	0.2	0.2	0.2	0.4	0.5	0.7	0.8
239.4	Neoplasm of unspecified nature of bladder	M	**0.2**	-	-	-	-	-	0.0	0.1	0.1	-
		F	**0.0**	-	-	-	-	-	-	-	-	-
239.6	Neoplasm of unspecified nature of brain	M	**0.7**	0.3	0.2	0.1	0.1	0.0	0.0	0.2	0.1	0.3
		F	**0.7**	0.3	0.1	-	0.1	0.1	0.1	0.1	0.2	0.3
239.7	Neoplasm of unspecified nature of other parts of nervous system and pituitary gland only	M	**0.1**	0.3	-	0.1	-	0.0	-	0.1	-	0.1
		F	**0.1**	-	-	0.1	-	0.1	0.1	0.1	0.1	0.1
630	Hydatidiform mole	F	**0.7**	-	-	-	-	1.4	2.2	2.9	2.0	0.4

40-44	45-49	50-54	55-59	60-64	65-69	70-74	75-79	80-84	85 and over		Site description	ICD (9th Revision) number
96.8	54.9	28.7	18.3	13.8	7.5	4.0	2.1	1.2	1.4	F	Carcinoma in situ of cervix uteri	233.1
-	-	-	-	0.2	0.2	0.1	-	-	-	M	Carcinoma in situ of other and	234
0.1	-	0.1	-	0.1	0.1	-	0.1	-	0.2	F	unspecified sites	
0.6	0.6	1.6	2.3	2.3	3.7	5.4	7.3	5.5	4.0	M	Neoplasm of uncertain behaviour of	235
1.0	1.2	1.5	2.3	2.5	3.8	5.1	4.7	4.6	3.5	F	digestive and respiratory systems	
0.4	1.0	1.3	2.0	3.3	2.7	4.7	4.5	6.4	9.3	M	Neoplasm of uncertain behaviour of	236
4.3	2.5	3.3	2.3	3.7	3.0	2.9	3.2	2.3	2.5	F	genitourinary organs	
0.6	0.7	1.0	1.0	1.2	1.6	1.0	1.4	0.9	1.3	M	Neoplasm of uncertain behaviour of	237
1.0	0.7	1.1	0.6	0.8	0.7	1.0	1.0	0.9	1.2	F	endocrine glands and nervous system	
1.0	1.4	1.8	3.8	4.8	6.6	10.6	12.3	17.2	14.7	M	Neoplasm of uncertain behaviour of	238
0.9	1.8	1.7	2.5	3.4	3.5	7.2	8.0	7.4	11.0	F	other and unspecified sites and tissues	
0.1	-	0.1	0.2	0.5	0.7	0.8	1.3	2.5	2.0	M	Neoplasm of unspecified nature of	239.4
-	-	0.1	0.1	0.1	-	-	0.2	0.3	0.2	F	bladder	
0.4	0.6	0.7	1.3	1.4	2.2	2.7	3.2	3.7	4.0	M	Neoplasm of unspecified nature of	239.6
0.3	0.2	0.6	0.5	0.8	1.7	2.2	3.5	2.3	4.7	F	brain	
0.1	0.1	-	0.2	0.5	0.6	0.3	0.2	-	1.3	M	Neoplasm of unspecified nature of	239.7
0.1	-	-	0.2	0.2	0.2	0.2	0.4	0.3	-	F	other parts of nervous system and pituitary gland only	
-	0.3	0.1	-	-	-	-	-	-	-	F	Hydatidiform mole	630

Table 6 All age crude rate and directly age - standardised rates per 100,000 population of newly diagnosed cases of cancer: sex and site, 1986

ICD (9th Revision) number	Site description	Crude rate M	Crude rate F	World standard population M	World standard population F	Truncated world standard population M	Truncated world standard population F	European standard population M	European standard population F	England and Wales 1981 standard population M	England and Wales 1981 standard population F
	All registrations	436.9	472.2	276.4	284.8	352.3	472.6	410.3	381.6	505.3	423.1
140-208	All malignant neoplasms	424.1	398.6	267.6	219.3	339.0	382.4	398.0	308.8	491.1	351.3
140	Malignant neoplasm of lip										
140.0	Upper lip, vermilion border	0.1	0.0	0.0	0.0	0.1	-	0.0	0.0	0.1	0.0
140.1	Lower lip, vermilion border	0.5	0.1	0.3	0.0	0.4	0.0	0.5	0.1	0.6	0.1
140.3	Upper lip, inner aspect	0.0	0.0	0.0	0.0	0.0	0.0	0.0	0.0	0.0	0.0
140.4	Lower lip, inner aspect	0.0	0.0	0.0	0.0	0.0	-	0.0	0.0	0.0	0.0
140.5	Lip, unspecified, inner aspect	0.0	-	0.0	-	-	-	0.0	-	0.0	-
140.6	Commissure of lip	-	0.0	-	0.0	-	-	-	0.0	-	0.0
140.8	Other	0.0	-	0.0	-	-	-	0.0	-	0.0	-
140.9	Lip, unspecified, vermilion border	0.2	0.0	0.1	0.0	0.1	0.0	0.2	0.0	0.2	0.0
141	Malignant neoplasm of tongue										
141.0	Base of tongue	0.3	0.1	0.2	0.1	0.4	0.1	0.3	0.1	0.3	0.1
141.1	Dorsal surface of tongue	0.0	0.0	0.0	0.0	0.0	-	0.0	0.0	0.0	0.0
141.2	Tip and lateral border of tongue	0.1	0.2	0.1	0.1	0.2	0.1	0.1	0.1	0.1	0.1
141.3	Ventral surface of tongue	0.0	0.0	0.0	0.0	0.0	0.0	0.0	0.0	0.0	0.0
141.4	Anterior two-thirds of tongue, part unspecified	0.1	0.0	0.0	0.0	0.1	-	0.1	0.0	0.1	0.0
141.5	Junctional zone	0.0	0.0	0.0	0.0	0.0	0.0	0.0	0.0	0.0	0.0
141.6	Lingual tonsil	0.0	0.0	0.0	0.0	0.1	-	0.0	0.0	0.0	0.0
141.8	Other	0.0	0.0	0.0	0.0	0.0	0.0	0.0	0.0	0.0	0.0
141.9	Tongue, unspecified	0.8	0.5	0.5	0.2	0.9	0.4	0.8	0.4	0.9	0.4
142	Malignant neoplasm of major salivary glands										
142.0	Parotid gland	0.5	0.4	0.3	0.3	0.4	0.5	0.5	0.4	0.6	0.4
142.1	Submandibular gland	0.1	0.1	0.1	0.1	0.1	0.1	0.1	0.1	0.1	0.1
142.2	Sublingual gland	0.0	0.0	0.0	0.0	0.0	0.0	0.0	0.0	0.0	0.0
142.8	Other	-	-	-	-	-	-	-	-	-	-
142.9	Site unspecified	0.0	0.1	0.0	0.0	0.0	0.0	0.0	0.0	0.1	0.1
143	Malignant neoplasm of gum										
143.0	Upper gum	0.1	0.0	0.0	0.0	0.0	0.0	0.0	0.0	0.1	0.0
143.1	Lower gum	0.1	0.1	0.1	0.0	0.1	0.0	0.1	0.0	0.1	0.0
143.8	Other	-	-	-	-	-	-	-	-	-	-
143.9	Gum, unspecified	0.1	0.1	0.1	0.1	0.2	0.1	0.1	0.1	0.2	0.1

Table 6 Crude and directly standardised rates - *continued*

ICD (9th Revision) number	Site description	Crude rate M	F	World standard population M	F	Truncated world standard population M	F	European standard population M	F	England and Wales 1981 standard population M	F
144	Malignant neoplasm of floor of mouth										
144.0	Anterior portion	0.0	0.0	0.0	0.0	0.1	-	0.0	0.0	0.1	0.0
144.1	Lateral portion	0.1	0.0	0.0	0.0	0.1	0.0	0.1	0.0	0.1	0.0
144.8	Other	0.0	0.0	0.0	0.0	0.0	0.0	0.0	0.0	0.0	0.0
144.9	Part unspecified	0.8	0.2	0.6	0.1	1.2	0.2	0.8	0.1	0.8	0.2
145	Malignant neoplasm of other and unspecified parts of mouth										
145.0	Cheek mucosa	0.2	0.1	0.1	0.1	0.2	0.1	0.2	0.1	0.2	0.1
145.1	Vestibule of mouth	0.0	0.0	0.0	0.0	0.0	0.0	0.0	0.0	0.0	0.0
145.2	Hard palate	0.0	0.1	0.0	0.0	0.1	0.1	0.0	0.0	0.0	0.0
145.3	Soft palate	0.2	0.1	0.1	0.1	0.2	0.1	0.1	0.1	0.2	0.1
145.4	Uvula	0.0	0.0	0.0	0.0	0.1	0.0	0.0	0.0	0.0	0.0
145.5	Palate, unspecified	0.1	0.0	0.1	0.0	0.1	0.0	0.1	0.0	0.1	0.0
145.6	Retromolar area	0.1	0.1	0.1	0.0	0.1	0.0	0.1	0.0	0.1	0.0
145.8	Other	0.0	0.0	0.0	0.0	0.0	0.0	0.0	0.0	0.0	0.0
145.9	Mouth, unspecified	0.2	0.1	0.1	0.1	0.2	0.1	0.2	0.1	0.2	0.1
146	Malignant neoplasm of oropharynx										
146.0	Tonsil	0.6	0.3	0.4	0.2	0.8	0.3	0.6	0.2	0.6	0.3
146.1	Tonsillar fossa	0.0	0.0	0.0	0.0	0.1	0.0	0.0	0.0	0.0	0.0
146.2	Tonsillar pillars (anterior) (posterior)	0.0	0.0	0.0	0.0	0.0	-	0.0	0.0	0.0	0.0
146.3	Vallecula	0.0	0.0	0.0	0.0	0.1	0.0	0.0	0.0	0.1	0.0
146.4	Anterior aspect of epiglottis	0.0	0.0	0.0	0.0	0.0	-	0.0	0.0	0.0	0.0
146.5	Junctional region	-	-	-	-	-	-	-	-	-	-
146.6	Lateral wall of oropharynx	0.0	-	0.0	-	0.0	-	0.0	-	0.0	-
146.7	Posterior wall of oropharynx	-	-	-	-	-	-	-	-	-	-
146.8	Other	0.0	0.0	0.0	0.0	0.0	0.0	0.0	0.0	0.0	0.0
146.9	Oropharynx, unspecified	0.2	0.1	0.1	0.0	0.3	0.1	0.2	0.1	0.2	0.1
147	Malignant neoplasm of nasopharynx										
147.0	Superior wall	-	-	-	-	-	-	-	-	-	-
147.1	Posterior wall	0.0	0.0	0.0	0.0	0.0	0.0	0.0	0.0	0.0	0.0
147.2	Lateral wall	0.0	-	0.0	-	0.0	-	0.0	-	0.0	-
147.3	Anterior wall	0.0	0.0	0.0	0.0	0.0	0.0	0.0	0.0	0.0	0.0
147.8	Other	0.0	0.0	0.0	0.0	-	-	0.0	0.0	0.0	0.0
147.9	Nasopharynx, unspecified	0.4	0.2	0.3	0.1	0.6	0.3	0.4	0.2	0.4	0.2

Table 6 Series MB1 no. 19

Table 6 Crude and directly standardised rates - *continued*

ICD (9th Revision) number	Site description	Crude rate M	Crude rate F	World standard population M	World standard population F	Truncated world standard population M	Truncated world standard population F	European standard population M	European standard population F	England and Wales 1981 standard population M	England and Wales 1981 standard population F
148	Malignant neoplasm of hypopharynx										
148.0	Postcricoid region	0.2	0.3	0.1	0.1	0.2	0.2	0.2	0.2	0.2	0.2
148.1	Pyriform sinus	0.6	0.2	0.4	0.1	0.7	0.2	0.5	0.1	0.6	0.2
148.2	Aryepiglottic fold, hypopharyngeal aspect	*0.0*	*0.0*	*0.0*	*0.0*	*0.0*	*0.0*	*0.0*	*0.0*	*0.0*	*0.0*
148.3	Posterior hypopharyngeal wall	*0.0*	*0.0*	*0.0*	*0.0*	*0.0*	-	*0.0*	*0.0*	*0.0*	*0.0*
148.8	Other	*0.0*	-	*0.0*	-	-	-	*0.0*	-	*0.0*	-
148.9	Hypopharynx, unspecified	0.1	*0.1*	0.1	0.0	0.1	0.0	0.1	0.0	0.1	*0.1*
149	Malignant neoplasm of other and ill-defined sites within the lip oral cavity and pharynx										
149.0	Pharynx, unspecified	0.3	0.2	0.2	0.1	0.4	0.2	0.3	0.1	0.4	0.1
149.1	Waldeyer's ring	-	-	-	-	-	-	-	-	-	-
149.8	Other	*0.0*	-	*0.0*	-	*0.0*	-	*0.0*	-	*0.0*	-
149.9	Ill-defined	*0.0*	*0.0*	*0.0*	*0.0*	*0.0*	-	*0.0*	*0.0*	*0.0*	*0.0*
150	Malignant neoplasm of oesophagus										
150.0	Cervical part	*0.0*	*0.0*	*0.0*	*0.0*	*0.0*	-	*0.0*	*0.0*	*0.0*	*0.0*
150.1	Thoracic part	*0.0*	*0.0*	*0.0*	*0.0*	*0.0*	-	*0.0*	*0.0*	*0.0*	*0.0*
150.2	Abdominal part	*0.0*	*0.0*	*0.0*	*0.0*	*0.0*	-	*0.0*	*0.0*	*0.0*	*0.0*
150.3	Upper third	0.3	0.3	0.2	0.1	0.2	0.2	0.3	0.2	0.3	0.3
150.4	Middle third	0.8	0.8	0.5	0.4	0.7	0.6	0.7	0.6	0.9	0.7
150.5	Lower third	2.9	1.5	1.8	0.7	2.6	0.9	2.7	1.0	3.3	1.3
150.8	Other	*0.0*	*0.0*	*0.0*	*0.0*	*0.0*	*0.0*	*0.0*	*0.0*	*0.0*	*0.0*
150.9	Oesophagus, unspecified	6.6	4.4	4.1	1.8	5.4	2.1	6.2	2.8	7.7	3.6
151	Malignant neoplasm of stomach										
151.0	Cardia	3.9	1.2	2.5	0.6	4.0	0.8	3.7	0.8	4.4	1.0
151.1	Pylorus	0.5	0.4	0.3	0.2	0.5	0.2	0.5	0.3	0.6	0.3
151.2	Pyloric antrum	1.5	1.2	0.9	0.5	1.1	0.6	1.4	0.8	1.7	1.0
151.3	Fundus of stomach	0.4	0.2	0.3	0.1	0.3	0.1	0.4	0.1	0.5	0.2
151.4	Body of stomach	0.7	0.4	0.4	0.1	0.5	0.2	0.6	0.2	0.8	0.3
151.5	Lesser curvature, unspecified	1.5	0.8	0.9	0.4	1.0	0.6	1.4	0.6	1.7	0.7
151.6	Greater curvature, unspecified	0.5	0.2	0.3	0.1	0.3	0.1	0.4	0.2	0.5	0.2
151.8	Other	0.5	0.3	0.3	0.1	0.4	0.2	0.5	0.2	0.6	0.2
151.9	Stomach, unspecified	17.6	10.9	10.4	4.2	11.1	4.0	16.3	6.7	20.9	8.6
152	Malignant neoplasm of small intestine, including duodenum										
152.0	Duodenum	0.1	0.2	0.1	0.1	0.1	0.2	0.1	0.1	0.2	0.2
152.1	Jejunum	0.1	*0.1*	0.1	0.0	0.2	*0.1*	0.1	*0.1*	0.1	*0.1*

Table 6 Crude and directly standardised rates - *continued*

ICD (9th Revision) number	Site description	Crude rate M	Crude rate F	World standard population M	World standard population F	Truncated world standard population M	Truncated world standard population F	European standard population M	European standard population F	England and Wales 1981 standard population M	England and Wales 1981 standard population F
152.2	Ileum	0.1	0.1	0.1	0.1	0.1	0.1	0.1	0.1	0.1	0.1
152.3	Meckel's diverticulum	*0.0*	*0.0*	*0.0*	*0.0*	*0.0*	-	*0.0*	*0.0*	*0.0*	*0.0*
152.8	Other	*0.0*	*0.0*	*0.0*	*0.0*	*0.0*	*0.0*	*0.0*	*0.0*	*0.0*	*0.0*
152.9	Small intestine, unspecified	0.3	0.2	0.2	0.1	0.3	0.2	0.3	0.2	0.3	0.2
153	Malignant neoplasm of colon										
153.0	Hepatic flexure	0.7	0.7	0.4	0.3	0.7	0.4	0.7	0.5	0.8	0.6
153.1	Transverse colon	1.7	2.2	1.1	1.0	1.4	1.5	1.6	1.6	2.0	1.9
153.2	Descending colon	1.3	1.2	0.8	0.6	1.0	1.0	1.2	0.9	1.5	1.1
153.3	Sigmoid colon	8.0	8.4	4.9	4.2	6.2	7.1	7.5	6.2	9.4	7.3
153.4	Caecum	4.6	6.9	2.8	2.8	3.0	3.3	4.3	4.4	5.5	5.5
153.5	Appendix	0.1	0.1	0.1	0.1	0.1	0.2	0.1	0.1	0.1	0.1
153.6	Ascending colon	2.0	2.2	1.2	1.0	1.4	1.5	1.9	1.5	2.4	1.8
153.7	Splenic flexure	0.8	0.9	0.5	0.4	0.6	0.6	0.8	0.6	1.0	0.7
153.8	Other	0.2	0.2	0.1	0.1	0.1	0.1	0.2	0.1	0.2	0.2
153.9	Colon, unspecified	7.4	9.2	4.5	3.9	5.5	5.1	7.0	6.0	8.7	7.4
154	Malignant neoplasm of rectum, rectosigmoid junction and anus										
154.0	Rectosigmoid junction	3.1	2.8	1.9	1.4	2.5	2.1	2.9	2.0	3.6	2.4
154.1	Rectum	17.3	12.6	10.8	5.8	14.6	8.2	16.3	8.7	20.1	10.6
154.2	Anal canal	0.3	0.4	0.2	0.2	0.3	0.4	0.3	0.3	0.4	0.4
154.3	Anus, unspecified	0.3	0.3	0.2	0.1	0.2	0.2	0.2	0.2	0.3	0.3
154.8	Other	0.1	*0.1*	0.1	0.0	0.1	*0.1*	0.1	0.0	0.1	*0.1*
155	Malignant neoplasm of liver and intrahepatic bile-ducts										
155.0	Liver, primary	2.1	1.2	1.4	0.6	2.0	0.8	2.0	0.9	2.4	1.0
155.1	Intrahepatic bile ducts	0.2	0.2	0.1	0.1	0.1	0.1	0.2	0.1	0.2	0.2
155.2	Liver, not specified as primary or secondary	0.2	0.1	0.1	0.0	0.1	0.1	0.2	0.1	0.2	0.1
156	Malignant neoplasm of gallbladder and extrahepatic bile ducts										
156.0	Gallbladder	0.7	1.5	0.4	0.6	0.4	0.8	0.6	1.0	0.8	1.2
156.1	Extrahepatic bile ducts	0.9	0.8	0.6	0.4	0.7	0.5	0.9	0.6	1.1	0.7
156.2	Ampulla of Vater	0.3	0.3	0.2	0.1	0.3	0.2	0.3	0.2	0.3	0.3
156.8	Other	*0.0*	*0.0*	*0.0*	*0.0*	-	*0.0*	*0.0*	*0.0*	*0.0*	*0.0*
156.9	Biliary ract, part unspecified	*0.1*	*0.1*	*0.0*	*0.0*	*0.1*	*0.0*	*0.1*	*0.0*	*0.1*	*0.0*
157	Malignant neoplasm of pancreas										
157.0	Head of pancreas	5.2	5.1	3.2	2.1	4.2	2.2	4.9	3.3	6.1	4.2
157.1	Body of pancreas	0.4	0.5	0.3	0.2	0.3	0.4	0.4	0.4	0.5	0.4

Table 6 Crude and directly standardised rates - *continued*

ICD (9th Revision) number	Site description	Crude rate M	Crude rate F	World standard population M	World standard population F	Truncated world standard population M	Truncated world standard population F	European standard population M	European standard population F	England and Wales 1981 standard population M	England and Wales 1981 standard population F
157.2	Tail of pancreas	0.2	0.2	0.1	0.1	0.1	0.2	0.2	0.2	0.3	0.2
157.3	Pancreatic duct	0.0	0.0	0.0	0.0	0.0	0.0	0.0	0.0	0.0	0.0
157.4	Islets of Langerhans	0.0	0.0	0.0	0.0	-	0.0	0.0	0.0	0.0	0.0
157.8	Other	0.1	0.1	0.1	0.1	0.1	0.1	0.1	0.1	0.1	0.1
157.9	Part unspecified	5.3	5.1	3.3	2.1	4.1	2.5	5.0	3.3	6.2	4.2
158	Malignant neoplasm of retroperitoneum and peritoneum										
158.0	Retroperitoneum	0.2	0.3	0.2	0.2	0.2	0.3	0.2	0.2	0.3	0.3
158.8	Specified parts of peritoneum	0.1	0.1	0.1	0.1	0.1	0.1	0.1	0.1	0.1	0.1
158.9	Peritoneum, unspecified	0.1	0.1	0.1	0.0	0.2	0.1	0.1	0.1	0.1	0.1
159	Malignant neoplasm of other and ill-defined sites within the digestive organs and peritoneum										
159.0	Intestinal tract, part unspecified	0.3	0.4	0.2	0.2	0.2	0.1	0.3	0.3	0.4	0.3
159.1	Spleen, not elsewhere classified	0.0	0.0	0.0	0.0	-	0.0	0.0	0.0	0.0	0.0
159.8	Other	0.0	0.0	0.0	0.0	0.0	0.0	0.0	0.0	0.0	0.0
159.9	Ill-defined	0.3	0.3	0.2	0.1	0.3	0.1	0.3	0.2	0.4	0.2
160	Malignant neoplasm of nasal cavities, middle ear and accessory sinuses										
160.0	Nasal cavities	0.3	0.2	0.2	0.1	0.3	0.2	0.3	0.2	0.3	0.2
160.1	Auditory tube, middle ear and mastoid air cells	0.1	0.1	0.1	0.0	0.1	0.1	0.1	0.0	0.1	0.0
160.2	Maxillary sinus	0.4	0.3	0.2	0.2	0.4	0.2	0.4	0.2	0.4	0.3
160.3	Ethmoidal sinus	0.1	0.0	0.0	0.0	0.0	0.0	0.1	0.0	0.1	0.0
160.4	Frontal sinus	0.0	0.0	0.0	0.0	-	0.0	0.0	0.0	0.0	0.0
160.5	Sphenoidal sinus	0.0	-	0.0	-	0.0	-	0.0	-	0.0	-
160.8	Other	0.0	0.0	0.0	0.0	0.0	-	0.0	0.0	0.0	0.0
160.9	Accessory sinus, unspecified	0.0	0.0	0.0	0.0	0.0	0.0	0.0	0.0	0.0	0.0
161	Malignant neoplasm of larynx										
161.0	Glottis	2.9	0.4	2.0	0.2	3.7	0.5	2.8	0.3	3.2	0.4
161.1	Supraglottis	0.9	0.3	0.6	0.2	0.9	0.4	0.8	0.2	1.0	0.3
161.2	Subglottis	0.1	0.1	0.1	0.0	0.0	0.1	0.1	0.1	0.1	0.1
161.3	Laryngeal cartilages	0.0	0.0	0.0	0.0	0.0	0.0	0.0	0.0	0.0	0.0
161.8	Other	0.0	0.0	0.0	0.0	-	-	0.0	0.0	0.0	0.0
161.9	Larynx, unspecified	2.1	0.5	1.4	0.3	2.3	0.5	2.0	0.4	2.4	0.4

Table 6 Crude and directly standardised rates - *continued*

ICD (9th Revision) number	Site description	Crude rate M	Crude rate F	World standard population M	World standard population F	Truncated world standard population M	Truncated world standard population F	European standard population M	European standard population F	England and Wales 1981 standard population M	England and Wales 1981 standard population F
162	Malignant neoplasm of trachea, bronchus and lung										
162.0	Trachea	0.2	0.2	0.2	0.1	0.3	0.2	0.2	0.1	0.3	0.1
162.2	Main bronchus	8.4	3.6	5.3	1.9	7.6	3.2	7.8	2.7	9.5	3.2
162.3	Upper lobe, bronchus or lung	20.2	7.7	12.7	4.4	18.2	7.8	18.6	6.2	22.9	7.2
162.4	Middle lobe, bronchus or lung	2.4	1.1	1.5	0.6	1.9	0.9	2.3	0.8	2.8	1.0
162.5	Lower lobe, bronchus or lung	11.0	3.8	6.8	2.0	8.8	3.2	10.1	2.9	12.6	3.4
162.8	Other	0.7	0.3	0.4	0.2	0.6	0.4	0.6	0.3	0.7	0.3
162.9	Bronchus and lung, unspecified	57.0	22.3	34.2	10.9	38.6	15.9	52.6	16.0	67.0	19.5
163	Malignant neoplasm of pleura										
163.0	Parietal	*0.0*	-	*0.0*	-	*0.0*	-	*0.0*	-	*0.0*	-
163.1	Visceral	-	-	-	-	-	-	-	-	-	-
163.8	Other	*0.0*	*0.0*	*0.0*	*0.0*	*0.0*	*0.0*	*0.0*	*0.0*	*0.0*	*0.0*
163.9	Pleura, unspecified	2.0	0.4	1.4	0.2	2.6	0.4	2.0	0.3	2.2	0.3
164	Malignant neoplasm of thymus heart and mediastinum										
164.0	Thymus	0.1	*0.1*	0.1	0.0	0.1	*0.1*	0.1	*0.1*	0.1	*0.1*
164.1	Heart	*0.0*	*0.0*	*0.0*	*0.0*	*0.0*	*0.0*	*0.0*	*0.0*	*0.0*	*0.0*
164.2	Anterior mediastinum	*0.0*	*0.0*	*0.0*	*0.0*	*0.0*	*0.0*	*0.0*	*0.0*	*0.0*	*0.0*
164.3	Posterior mediastinum	*0.0*	*0.0*	*0.0*	*0.0*	*0.0*	-	*0.0*	*0.0*	*0.0*	*0.0*
164.8	Other	*0.0*	*0.0*	*0.0*	*0.0*	*0.0*	-	*0.0*	*0.0*	*0.0*	*0.0*
164.9	Mediastinum, part unspecified	0.2	0.1	0.1	0.1	0.2	0.1	0.2	0.1	0.2	0.1
165	Malignant neoplasm of other and ill-defined sites within the respiratory system and intrathoracic organs										
165.0	Upper respiratory tract, part unspecified	*0.0*	-	*0.0*	-	-	-	*0.0*	-	*0.0*	-
165.8	Other	*0.0*	-	*0.0*	-	-	-	*0.0*	-	*0.0*	-
165.9	Ill-defined sites within the respiratory system	*0.0*	*0.0*	*0.0*	*0.0*	*0.0*	-	*0.0*	*0.0*	*0.0*	*0.0*
170	Malignant neoplasm of bone and articular cartilage										
170.0	Bones of skull and face	*0.1*	*0.1*	*0.1*	*0.0*	*0.1*	*0.0*	*0.1*	*0.1*	*0.1*	*0.1*
170.1	Lower jaw bone	*0.1*	*0.1*	*0.1*	*0.0*	*0.1*	*0.1*	*0.1*	*0.0*	*0.1*	*0.1*
170.2	Vertebral column, excluding sacrum and coccyx	0.1	0.1	0.1	0.1	0.1	0.1	0.1	0.1	0.1	0.1
170.3	Ribs, sternum and clavicle	*0.0*	*0.0*	*0.0*	*0.0*	*0.0*	*0.0*	*0.0*	*0.0*	*0.0*	*0.0*
170.4	Long bones of upper limb and scapula	0.1	*0.1*	0.1	*0.1*	0.1	*0.1*	0.1	*0.1*	0.1	*0.1*
170.5	Upper limb, short bones	*0.0*	*0.0*	*0.0*	*0.0*	*0.1*	-	*0.0*	*0.0*	*0.0*	*0.0*

Table 6 Crude and directly standardised rates - *continued*

ICD (9th Revision) number	Site description	Crude rate M	Crude rate F	World standard population M	World standard population F	Truncated world standard population M	Truncated world standard population F	European standard population M	European standard population F	England and Wales 1981 standard population M	England and Wales 1981 standard population F
170.6	Pelvic bones, sacrum and coccyx	0.2	0.1	0.1	0.1	0.2	0.1	0.2	0.1	0.2	0.1
170.7	Lower limb, long bones	0.3	0.2	0.2	0.3	0.2	0.1	0.2	0.2	0.3	0.2
170.8	Lower limb, short bones	0.0	0.0	0.0	0.0	0.0	0.0	0.0	0.0	0.0	0.0
170.9	Site unspecified	0.1	0.1	0.1	0.1	0.0	0.1	0.1	0.1	0.1	0.1
171	Malignant neoplasm of connective and other soft tissue										
171.0	Head, face and neck	0.1	0.1	0.1	0.1	0.1	0.1	0.2	0.1	0.2	0.1
171.2	Upper limb, including shoulder	0.3	0.2	0.2	0.1	0.4	0.2	0.3	0.2	0.3	0.2
171.3	Lower limb, including hip	0.6	0.6	0.4	0.4	0.6	0.6	0.6	0.5	0.6	0.5
171.4	Thorax	0.1	0.1	0.1	0.1	0.2	0.1	0.1	0.1	0.2	0.1
171.5	Abdomen	0.2	0.2	0.1	0.1	0.2	0.2	0.2	0.2	0.2	0.2
171.6	Pelvis	0.2	0.2	0.2	0.1	0.3	0.2	0.2	0.2	0.2	0.2
171.7	Trunk unspecified	0.1	0.0	0.1	0.0	0.1	0.0	0.1	0.0	0.1	0.0
171.8	Other	0.0	0.0	0.0	0.0	0.0	0.1	0.0	0.0	0.0	0.0
171.9	Site unspecified	0.2	0.2	0.1	0.2	0.2	0.2	0.2	0.2	0.2	0.2
172	Malignant melanoma of skin										
172.0	lip	0.0	0.0	0.0	0.0	-	0.0	0.0	0.0	0.0	0.0
172.1	Eyelid, including canthus	0.0	0.0	0.0	0.0	0.0	0.0	0.0	0.0	0.0	0.0
172.2	Ear and external auricular canal	0.1	0.0	0.1	0.0	0.1	0.0	0.1	0.0	0.1	0.0
172.3*	Other and unspecified parts of face	0.5	0.7	0.3	0.3	0.4	0.5	0.5	0.5	0.6	0.6
172.4	Scalp and neck	0.2	0.2	0.2	0.1	0.3	0.2	0.2	0.2	0.3	0.2
172.5	Trunk, except scrotum	1.4	0.9	1.1	0.8	2.4	1.5	1.4	0.9	1.4	0.9
172.6	Upper limb, including shoulder	0.7	1.2	0.5	0.9	1.2	1.9	0.7	1.1	0.7	1.2
172.7	Lower limb, including hip	0.7	3.4	0.5	2.6	1.0	5.2	0.7	3.2	0.7	3.3
172.8	Other	0.0	0.0	0.0	0.0	0.0	0.1	0.0	0.0	0.0	0.0
172.9	Site unspecified	0.5	0.5	0.4	0.4	0.7	0.8	0.5	0.5	0.5	0.5
173	Other malignant neoplasm of skin										
173.0	Skin of lip	1.6	1.3	1.0	0.6	1.5	1.0	1.5	0.9	1.8	1.1
173.1	Eyelid, including canthus	4.9	4.7	3.1	2.5	4.9	4.4	4.6	3.6	5.6	4.1
173.2	Ear and external auricular canal	6.2	1.0	3.7	0.5	3.4	0.5	5.8	0.7	7.5	0.9
173.3	Skin of other and unspecified parts of face	27.2	26.1	17.3	12.4	25.0	18.2	25.9	18.3	31.4	22.0
173.4	Scalp and skin of neck	4.6	3.5	2.9	1.6	3.4	2.1	4.4	2.4	5.5	2.9
173.5	Skin of trunk, except scrotum	3.7	2.7	2.5	1.5	4.6	2.6	3.6	2.1	4.1	2.4

Table 6 Crude and directly standardised rates - *continued*

ICD (9th Revision) number	Site description	Crude rate M	Crude rate F	World standard population M	World standard population F	Truncated world standard population M	Truncated world standard population F	European standard population M	European standard population F	England and Wales 1981 standard population M	England and Wales 1981 standard population F
173.6	Skin of upper limb, including shoulder	3.3	1.8	2.1	0.8	3.0	1.2	3.1	1.2	3.8	1.5
173.7	Skin of lower limb, including hip	1.4	3.9	0.8	1.9	1.2	2.8	1.2	2.8	1.5	3.4
173.8	Other	1.4	1.0	0.9	0.4	1.0	0.5	1.4	0.6	1.7	0.8
173.9	Site unspecified	3.7	3.2	2.4	1.6	3.6	2.6	3.5	2.3	4.2	2.7
174	Malignant neoplasm of female breast										
174.0	Nipple and areola	-	1.1	-	0.6	-	1.3	-	0.9	-	1.0
174.1	Central portion	-	3.0	-	2.0	-	4.5	-	2.7	-	2.8
174.2	Upper - inner quadrant	-	4.2	-	2.9	-	6.9	-	3.9	-	4.0
174.3	Lower - inner quadrant	-	1.8	-	1.2	-	2.9	-	1.7	-	1.7
174.4	Upper - outer quadrant	-	14.7	-	9.9	-	22.5	-	13.3	-	13.8
174.5	Lower - outer quadrant	-	2.7	-	1.8	-	4.3	-	2.5	-	2.6
174.6	Axillary tail	-	0.6	-	0.4	-	0.9	-	0.5	-	0.5
174.8	Other	-	5.1	-	3.5	-	8.1	-	4.7	-	4.9
174.9	Breast, unspecified	-	55.4	-	34.6	-	75.7	-	47.5	-	50.4
175	Malignant neoplasm of male breast	0.6	-	0.4	-	0.7	-	0.6	-	0.7	-
179	Malignant neoplasm of uterus, part unspecified	-	1.5	-	0.8	-	1.5	-	1.2	-	1.3
180	Malignant neoplasm of cervix uteri										
180.0	Endocervix	-	0.9	-	0.6	-	1.3	-	0.8	-	0.8
180.1	Exocervix	-	*0.1*	-	*0.0*	-	*0.1*	-	*0.1*	-	*0.1*
180.8	Other	-	0.1	-	0.1	-	0.2	-	0.1	-	0.1
180.9	Cervix uteri, unspecified	-	14.7	-	11.2	-	23.0	-	14.0	-	14.0
181	Malignant neoplasm of placenta	-	*0.0*	-	*0.0*	-	*0.0*	-	*0.0*	-	*0.0*
182	Malignant neoplasm of body of uterus										
182.0	Corpus uteri, except isthmus	-	13.4	-	7.9	-	16.6	-	11.3	-	12.4
182.1	Isthmus	-	*0.0*	-	*0.0*	-	*0.0*	-	*0.0*	-	*0.0*
182.8	Other	-	*0.0*	-	*0.0*	-	-	-	*0.0*	-	*0.0*
183	Malignant neoplasm of ovary and other uterine adnexa										
183.0	Ovary	-	17.4	-	10.9	-	22.6	-	15.0	-	16.2
183.2	Fallopian tube	-	0.1	-	0.1	-	0.2	-	0.1	-	0.1
183.3	Broad ligament	-	*0.0*	-	*0.0*	-	-	-	*0.0*	-	*0.0*
183.4	Parametrium	-	*0.0*	-	*0.0*	-	*0.0*	-	*0.0*	-	*0.0*
183.5	Round ligament	-	-	-	-	-	-	-	-	-	-
183.8	Other	-	*0.0*	-	*0.0*	-	*0.0*	-	*0.0*	-	*0.0*
183.9	Uterine adnexa, unspecified	-	*0.0*	-	*0.0*	-	-	-	*0.0*	-	*0.0*

Table 6 Crude and directly standardised rates - *continued*

ICD (9th Revision) number	Site description	Crude rate M	Crude rate F	World standard population M	World standard population F	Truncated world standard population M	Truncated world standard population F	European standard population M	European standard population F	England and Wales 1981 standard population M	England and Wales 1981 standard population F
184	Malignant neoplasm of other and unspecified female genital organs										
184.0	Vagina	-	0.7	-	0.3	-	0.5	-	0.5	-	0.6
184.1	Labia majora	-	0.1	-	0.1	-	0.1	-	0.1	-	0.1
184.2	Labia minora	-	0.0	-	0.0	-	0.0	-	0.0	-	0.0
184.3	Clitoris	-	0.0	-	0.0	-	0.0	-	0.0	-	0.0
184.4	Vulva, unspecified	-	2.8	-	1.2	-	1.3	-	1.8	-	2.3
184.8	Other	-	0.0	-	0.0	-	0.0	-	0.0	-	0.0
184.9	Site unspecified	-	0.1	-	0.1	-	0.2	-	0.1	-	0.1
185	Malignant neoplasm of prostate	41.7	-	23.0	-	13.3	-	37.8	-	51.2	-
186	Malignant neoplasm of testis										
186.0	Undescended	0.0	-	0.0	-	0.0	-	0.0	-	0.0	-
186.9	Other and unspecified	4.1	-	3.8	-	5.0	-	4.0	-	3.9	-
187	Malignant neoplasm of penis and other male genital organs										
187.1	Prepuce	0.1	-	0.1	-	0.1	-	0.1	-	0.1	-
187.2	Glans penis	0.2	-	0.1	-	0.1	-	0.2	-	0.2	-
187.3	Body of penis	0.0	-	0.0	-	0.0	-	0.0	-	0.0	-
187.4	Penis, part unspecified	0.8	-	0.5	-	0.6	-	0.7	-	0.9	-
187.5	Epididymis	0.0	-	0.0	-	-	-	0.0	-	0.0	-
187.6	Spermatic cord	0.0	-	0.0	-	0.0	-	0.0	-	0.0	-
187.7	Scrotum	0.2	-	0.1	-	0.1	-	0.2	-	0.2	-
187.8	Other	0.0	-	0.0	-	-	-	0.0	-	0.0	-
187.9	Site unspecified	0.0	-	0.0	-	0.0	-	0.0	-	0.0	-
188	Malignant neoplasm of bladder										
188.0	Trigone	0.1	0.0	0.0	0.0	0.0	-	0.1	0.0	0.1	0.0
188.1	Dome	0.0	0.0	0.0	0.0	0.0	-	0.0	0.0	0.1	0.0
188.2	Lateral wall	0.5	0.2	0.3	.1	0.4	0.2	0.5	0.2	0.6	0.2
188.3	Anterior wall	0.1	0.0	0.1	0.0	0.1	0.0	0.1	0.0	0.1	0.0
188.4	Posterior wall	0.1	0.0	0.1	0.0	0.1	0.0	0.1	0.0	0.1	0.0
188.5	Bladder neck	0.3	0.1	0.2	0.0	0.2	0.0	0.2	0.0	0.3	0.1
188.6	Ureteric orifice	0.4	0.2	0.3	0.1	0.4	0.2	0.4	0.1	0.4	0.1
188.7	Urachus	0.0	0.0	0.0	0.0	0.0	0.0	0.0	0.0	0.0	0.0
188.8	Other	0.6	0.2	0.4	0.1	0.4	0.1	0.5	0.2	0.7	0.2
188.9	Part unspecified	25.7	10.1	15.8	4.7	19.9	6.5	24.0	7.0	29.9	8.6

Table 6 Crude and directly standardised rates - *continued*

ICD (9th Revision) number	Site description	Crude rate M	Crude rate F	World standard population M	World standard population F	Truncated world standard population M	Truncated world standard population F	European standard population M	European standard population F	England and Wales 1981 standard population M	England and Wales 1981 standard population F
189	Malignant neoplasm of kidney and other and unspecified urinary organs										
189.0	Kidney except pelvis	6.6	3.9	4.5	2.3	7.7	3.8	6.4	3.1	7.4	3.5
189.1	Renal pelvis	0.5	0.3	0.4	0.2	0.7	0.3	0.5	0.2	0.6	0.3
189.2	Ureter	0.4	0.2	0.3	0.1	0.4	0.1	0.4	0.2	0.5	0.2
189.3	Urethra	0.1	0.1	0.1	0.0	0.0	0.1	0.1	0.1	0.1	0.1
189.4	Paraurethral glands	-	-	-	-	-	-	-	-	-	-
189.8	Other	*0.0*	*0.0*	*0.0*	*0.0*	*0.0*	*0.0*	*0.0*	*0.0*	*0.0*	*0.0*
189.9	Site unspecified	*0.1*	*0.1*	*0.0*	*0.0*	*0.0*	*0.0*	*0.1*	*0.0*	*0.1*	*0.0*
190	Malignant neoplasm of eye										
190.0	Eyeball, except conjunctiva, cornea, retina and choroid	*0.1*	*0.0*	*0.1*	*0.0*	*0.1*	*0.0*	*0.1*	*0.0*	*0.1*	*0.0*
190.1	Orbit	*0.1*	*0.0*	*0.1*	*0.0*	*0.1*	*0.0*	*0.1*	*0.0*	*0.1*	*0.0*
190.2	Lacrimal gland	-	-	-	-	-	-	-	-	-	-
190.3	Conjunctiva	*0.0*	*0.0*	*0.0*	*0.0*	*0.0*	-	*0.0*	*0.0*	*0.0*	*0.0*
190.4	Cornea	*0.0*	*0.0*	*0.0*	*0.0*	-	*0.0*	*0.0*	*0.0*	*0.0*	*0.0*
190.5	Retina	*0.0*	*0.0*	*0.1*	*0.1*	-	-	*0.0*	*0.0*	*0.0*	*0.0*
190.6	Choroid	0.2	0.2	0.2	0.1	0.4	0.3	0.2	0.2	0.3	0.2
190.7	Lacrimal duct	*0.0*	-	*0.0*	-	-	-	*0.0*	-	*0.0*	-
190.8	Other	*0.0*	*0.0*	*0.0*	*0.0*	-	*0.0*	*0.0*	*0.0*	*0.0*	*0.0*
190.9	Part unspecified	0.3	0.2	0.2	0.1	0.3	0.2	0.3	0.2	0.3	0.2
191	Malignant neoplasm of brain										
191.0	Cerebrum, except lobes and ventricles	0.8	0.6	0.7	0.4	1.1	0.7	0.8	0.5	0.9	0.5
191.1	Frontal lobe	0.9	0.7	0.7	0.5	1.5	1.2	0.9	0.7	0.9	0.7
191.2	Temporal lobe	0.7	0.4	0.6	0.3	1.1	0.6	0.7	0.4	0.7	0.4
191.3	Parietal lobe	0.9	0.6	0.7	0.4	1.5	0.9	0.9	0.6	1.0	0.6
191.4	Occipital lobe	0.2	*0.1*	0.2	*0.1*	0.2	*0.1*	0.2	*0.1*	0.2	*0.1*
191.5	Ventricle	0.1	0.1	0.1	0.1	0.1	0.0	0.1	0.1	0.1	0.1
191.6	Cerebellum	0.2	0.1	0.2	0.1	0.2	0.1	0.2	0.1	0.2	0.1
191.7	Brain stem	0.1	0.1	0.1	0.1	0.1	0.1	0.1	0.1	0.1	0.1
191.8	Other	0.6	0.4	0.4	0.3	0.8	0.5	0.6	0.3	0.6	0.4
191.9	Brain, unspecified	1.7	1.2	1.4	1.0	2.5	1.6	1.7	1.2	1.8	1.2
192	Malignant neoplasm of other and unspecified parts of nervous system										
192.0	Cranial nerves	*0.0*	*0.0*	*0.0*	*0.1*	*0.0*	*0.0*	*0.0*	*0.0*	*0.0*	*0.0*
192.1	Cerebral meninges	*0.0*	*0.1*	*0.0*	*0.0*	*0.0*	*0.1*	*0.0*	*0.1*	*0.0*	*0.1*

Table 6 Crude and directly standardised rates - *continued*

ICD (9th Revision) number	Site description	Crude rate M	Crude rate F	World standard population M	World standard population F	Truncated world standard population M	Truncated world standard population F	European standard population M	European standard population F	England and Wales 1981 standard population M	England and Wales 1981 standard population F
192.2	Spinal cord	0.1	0.1	0.1	0.1	0.1	0.1	0.1	0.1	0.1	0.1
192.3	Spinal meninges	0.0	-	0.0	-	-	-	0.0	-	0.0	-
192.8	Other	0.0	0.0	0.0	0.0	-	0.0	0.0	0.0	0.0	0.0
192.9	Part unspecified	0.0	0.0	0.0	0.0	0.0	0.0	0.0	0.0	0.0	0.0
193	Malignant neoplasm of thyroid gland	0.9	2.0	0.6	1.5	1.0	2.5	0.9	1.8	1.0	1.9
194	Malignant neoplasm of other endocrine glands and related structures										
194.0	Suprarenal gland	0.2	0.2	0.2	0.2	0.2	0.1	0.2	0.2	0.2	0.2
194.1	Parathyroid gland	-	-	-	-	-	-	-	-	-	-
194.3	Pituitary gland and Craniopharyngeal duct	0.1	0.1	0.0	0.0	0.1	0.1	0.0	0.1	0.1	0.1
194.4	Pineal gland	0.0	0.0	0.0	0.0	0.0	0.0	0.0	0.0	0.0	0.0
194.5	Carotid body	-	0.0	-	0.0	-	-	-	0.0	-	0.0
194.6	Aortic body and other paraganglia	-	0.0	-	0.0	-	0.0	-	0.0	-	0.0
194.8	Other	-	-	-	-	-	-	-	-	-	-
194.9	Site unspecified	0.0	0.0	0.0	0.0	0.0	0.0	0.0	0.0	0.0	0.0
195	Malignant neoplasm of other and ill-defined sites										
195.0	Head, face and neck	0.1	0.1	0.1	0.1	0.2	0.1	0.1	0.1	0.2	0.1
195.1	Thorax	0.1	0.0	0.1	0.0	0.1	0.0	0.1	0.0	0.1	0.0
195.2	Abdomen	0.3	0.5	0.2	0.2	0.2	0.2	0.2	0.3	0.3	0.4
195.3	Pelvis	0.0	0.2	0.0	0.1	0.0	0.2	0.0	0.2	0.0	0.2
195.4	Upper limb	0.0	0.1	0.0	0.0	0.0	0.0	0.0	0.0	0.0	0.0
195.5	Lower limb	0.0	0.1	0.0	0.0	0.0	0.0	0.0	0.0	0.0	0.1
195.8	Other specified sites	0.0	-	0.0	-	0.0	-	0.0	-	0.0	-
196	Secondary and unspecified malignant neoplasm of lymph nodes										
196.0	Head, face and neck	0.7	0.5	0.5	0.3	0.8	0.5	0.7	0.4	0.8	0.4
196.1	Intrathoracic	0.0	0.0	0.0	0.0	0.0	0.0	0.0	0.0	0.0	0.0
196.2	Intra-abdominal	0.0	0.0	0.0	0.0	0.0	0.0	0.0	0.0	0.0	0.0
196.3	Axilla and upper limb	0.1	0.2	0.1	0.1	0.1	0.2	0.1	0.1	0.1	0.2
196.5	Inguinal and lower limb	0.1	0.1	0.1	0.0	0.1	0.1	0.1	0.1	0.1	0.1
196.6	Intrapelvic	0.0	0.0	0.0	0.0	0.0	-	0.0	0.0	0.0	0.0
196.8	Multiple sites	0.0	0.0	0.0	0.0	0.0	0.0	0.0	0.0	0.0	0.0
196.9	Site unspecified	0.2	0.2	0.2	0.1	0.3	0.2	0.2	0.2	0.3	0.2

Table 6 Crude and directly standardised rates - *continued*

ICD (9th Revision) number	Site description	Crude rate M	Crude rate F	World standard population M	World standard population F	Truncated world standard population M	Truncated world standard population F	European standard population M	European standard population F	England and Wales 1981 standard population M	England and Wales 1981 standard population F
197	Secondary malignant neoplasm of respiratory and digestive systems										
197.0	Lung	0.9	0.7	0.6	0.3	0.7	0.4	0.8	0.5	1.0	0.6
197.1	Mediastinum	*0.0*	*0.0*	*0.0*	*0.0*	*0.0*	*0.0*	*0.0*	*0.0*	*0.0*	*0.0*
197.2	Pleura	0.4	0.4	0.2	0.2	0.3	0.3	0.3	0.3	0.4	0.4
197.3	Other respiratory organs	*0.0*	*0.0*	*0.0*	*0.0*	*0.0*	-	*0.0*	*0.0*	*0.0*	*0.0*
197.4	Small intestine, including duodenum	*0.0*	*0.0*	*0.0*	*0.0*	-	*0.0*	*0.0*	*0.0*	*0.0*	*0.0*
197.5	Large intestine and rectum	*0.1*	0.1	*0.0*	0.0	*0.0*	0.1	*0.1*	0.1	*0.1*	0.1
197.6	Retroperitoneum and peritoneum	0.4	1.1	0.3	0.5	0.4	0.7	0.4	0.8	0.5	1.0
197.7	Liver	4.8	4.1	2.9	1.8	3.3	2.5	4.4	2.8	5.6	3.4
197.8	Other digestive organs	0.2	0.2	0.1	0.1	0.1	0.1	0.1	0.1	0.2	0.1
198	Secondary malignant neoplasm of other specified sites										
198.0	Kidney	*0.0*	*0.0*	*0.0*	*0.0*	*0.0*	*0.0*	*0.0*	*0.0*	*0.0*	*0.0*
198.1	Other urinary organs	*0.0*	*0.0*	*0.0*	*0.0*	*0.0*	-	*0.0*	*0.0*	*0.0*	*0.0*
198.2	Skin	0.2	0.2	0.1	0.1	0.2	0.1	0.2	0.1	0.2	0.2
198.3	Brain and spinal cord	1.0	0.7	0.7	0.4	1.2	0.9	0.9	0.6	1.1	0.7
198.4	Other parts of nervous system	*0.0*	*0.0*	*0.0*	*0.0*	*0.0*	-	*0.0*	*0.0*	*0.0*	*0.0*
198.5	Bone and bone marrow	1.6	1.3	1.0	0.6	1.2	0.9	1.5	0.9	1.8	1.1
198.6	Ovary	-	0.1	-	0.1	-	0.2	-	0.1	-	0.1
198.7	Suprarenal gland	*0.0*	*0.0*	*0.0*	*0.0*	-	-	*0.0*	*0.0*	*0.0*	*0.0*
198.8	Other specified sites	0.5	0.8	0.3	0.4	0.4	0.6	0.4	0.5	0.5	0.6
199	Malignant neoplasm without specification of site										
199.0	Disseminated	5.4	5.4	3.2	2.2	2.9	2.7	5.0	3.5	6.6	4.4
199.1	Other	4.1	4.3	2.5	1.8	2.7	2.1	3.9	2.8	4.9	3.4
200	Lymphosarcoma and reticulosarcoma										
200.0	Reticulosarcoma	0.2	0.1	0.1	0.1	0.2	0.1	0.2	0.1	0.2	0.1
200.1	Lymphosarcoma	0.8	0.6	0.6	0.3	0.8	0.6	0.8	0.5	0.9	0.5
200.2	Burkitt's Tumour	*0.0*	*0.0*	*0.0*	*0.0*	*0.0*	*0.0*	*0.0*	*0.0*	*0.0*	*0.0*
200.8	Other named variants	0.2	0.2	0.1	0.1	0.3	0.1	0.2	0.1	0.2	0.1
201	Hodgkin's disease										
201.0	Hodgkin's paragranuloma	*0.0*	-	*0.0*	-	-	-	*0.0*	-	*0.0*	-
201.1	Hodgkin's granuloma	-	-	-	-	-	-	-	-	-	-
201.2	Hodgkin's sarcoma	-	-	-	-	-	-	-	-	-	-
201.4	Lymphocytic-histiocytic predominance	0.2	*0.1*	0.2	0.0	0.2	*0.1*	0.2	0.0	0.2	*0.1*

Table 6 Series MB1 no. 19

Table 6 Crude and directly standardised rates - *continued*

ICD (9th Revision) number	Site description	Crude rate M	F	World standard population M	F	Truncated world standard population M	F	European standard population M	F	England and Wales 1981 standard population M	F
201.5	Nodular sclerosis	0.8	0.8	0.8	0.7	0.8	0.5	0.8	0.7	0.8	0.7
201.6	Mixed cellularity	0.5	0.3	0.4	0.2	0.5	0.3	0.5	0.2	0.5	0.3
201.7	Lymphocytic depletion	0.1	0.0	0.1	0.0	0.1	0.0	0.1	0.0	0.1	0.0
201.9	Unspecified	1.2	0.7	1.1	0.6	1.4	0.4	1.2	0.6	1.3	0.7
202	Other malignant neoplasm of lymphoid and histiocytic tissue										
202.0	Nodular nymphoma	0.6	0.7	0.4	0.5	1.0	0.9	0.6	0.6	0.6	0.7
202.1	Mycosis fungoides	0.2	0.1	0.1	0.1	0.1	0.1	0.1	0.1	0.2	0.1
202.2	Sezary's disease	0.0	0.0	0.0	0.0	0.0	-	0.0	0.0	0.0	0.0
202.3	Malignant histiocytosis	0.1	0.0	0.0	0.0	0.1	0.0	0.1	0.0	0.1	0.0
202.4	Leukaemic reticuloendotheliosis	0.2	0.0	0.2	0.0	0.4	0.1	0.2	0.0	0.2	0.0
202.5	Letterer-Siwe disease	0.0	-	0.0	-	-	-	0.0	-	0.0	-
202.6	Malignant mast-cell tumours	0.0	-	0.0	-	-	-	0.0	-	0.0	-
202.8	Other lymphomas	7.8	6.6	5.5	3.7	8.6	5.9	7.5	5.1	8.6	5.8
202.9	Other and unspecified	0.1	0.0	0.0	0.0	0.1	0.0	0.1	0.0	0.1	0.0
203	Multiple myeloma and immunoproliferative neoplasms										
203.0	Multiple Myeloma	4.7	3.9	2.9	1.8	3.7	2.4	4.4	2.7	5.5	3.3
203.1	Plasma cell leukaemia	0.0	0.0	0.0	0.0	0.0	0.0	0.0	0.0	0.0	0.0
203.8	Other immunoproliferative neoplasms	0.0	0.0	0.0	0.0	0.0	0.0	0.0	0.0	0.1	0.0
204	Lymphoid leukaemia										
204.0	Acute	1.1	0.8	1.4	1.0	0.5	0.3	1.2	0.8	1.2	0.8
204.1	Chronic	2.5	1.8	1.5	0.7	1.6	0.6	2.4	1.1	3.0	1.4
204.2	Subacute	-	-	-	-	-	-	-	-	-	-
204.8	Other	0.0	0.0	0.0	0.0	-	-	0.0	0.0	0.0	0.0
204.9	Unspecified	0.2	0.1	0.1	0.1	0.1	0.1	0.2	0.1	0.2	0.1
205	Myeloid leukaemia										
205.0	Acute	2.6	2.3	1.8	1.4	2.3	2.0	2.4	1.8	2.9	2.0
205.1	Chronic	1.3	1.1	0.8	0.5	1.1	0.8	1.2	0.8	1.5	0.9
205.2	Subacute	-	0.0	-	0.0	-	0.0	-	0.0	-	0.0
205.3	Myeloid sarcoma	0.0	-	0.0	-	-	-	0.0	-	0.0	-
205.8	Other	0.0	0.0	0.0	0.0	0.0	-	0.0	0.0	0.0	0.0
205.9	Unspecified	0.2	0.2	0.1	0.1	0.1	0.1	0.2	0.1	0.2	0.1
206	Monocytic leukaemia										
206.0	Acute	0.1	0.1	0.1	0.1	0.1	0.1	0.1	0.1	0.1	0.1
206.1	Chronic	0.0	0.0	0.0	0.0	-	-	0.0	0.0	0.0	0.0

Table 6 Crude and directly standardised rates - *continued*

ICD (9th Revision) number	Site description	Crude rate M	Crude rate F	World standard population M	World standard population F	Truncated world standard population M	Truncated world standard population F	European standard population M	European standard population F	England and Wales 1981 standard population M	England and Wales 1981 standard population F
206.2	Subacute	0.0	0.0	0.0	0.0	-	-	0.0	0.0	0.0	0.0
206.8	Other	-	0.0	-	0.0	-	-	-	0.0	-	0.0
206.9	Unspecified	0.0	0.0	0.0	0.0	0.0	-	0.0	0.0	0.0	0.0
207	Other specified leukaemia										
207.0	Acute erythraemia and erythroleukaemia	0.1	0.0	0.0	0.0	0.0	0.0	0.1	0.0	0.1	0.0
207.1	Chronic erythraemia	-	-	-	-	-	-	-	-	-	-
207.2	Megakaryocytic leukaemia	0.0	0.0	0.0	0.0	0.0	0.0	0.0	0.0	0.0	0.0
207.8	Other	0.0	0.0	0.0	0.0	-	-	0.0	0.0	0.0	0.0
208	Leukaemia of unspecified cell type										
208.0	Acute	0.2	0.2	0.1	0.1	0.2	0.1	0.2	0.2	0.2	0.2
208.1	Chronic	0.0	0.0	0.0	0.0	-	-	0.0	0.0	0.0	0.0
208.2	Subacute	-	0.0	-	0.0	-	-	-	0.0	-	0.0
208.8	Other	0.0	0.0	0.0	0.0	-	-	0.0	0.0	0.0	0.0
208.9	Unspecified	0.4	0.2	0.2	0.1	0.2	0.1	0.3	0.1	0.4	0.2
223.3	Benign neoplasm of bladder	0.1	0.1	0.1	0.0	0.1	0.1	0.1	0.1	0.1	0.1
225	Benign neoplasm of brain and other parts of nervous system										
225.0	Brain	0.2	0.2	0.1	0.2	0.1	0.4	0.2	0.2	0.2	0.2
225.1	Cranial nerves	0.2	0.3	0.2	0.3	0.4	0.5	0.2	0.3	0.2	0.3
225.2	Cerebral meninges	0.7	1.4	0.5	0.9	1.0	2.0	0.7	1.2	0.7	1.3
225.3	Spinal cord	0.1	0.1	0.1	0.1	0.1	0.1	0.1	0.1	0.1	0.1
225.4	Spinal meninges	0.0	0.1	0.0	0.1	0.0	0.1	0.0	0.1	0.0	0.1
225.8	Other	0.0	0.0	0.0	0.0	0.0	-	0.0	0.0	0.0	0.0
225.9	Part unspecified	0.0	0.0	0.0	0.0	0.0	0.1	0.0	0.0	0.0	0.0
227.3	Benign neoplasm of pituitary gland and craniopharyngeal duct	0.7	0.6	0.5	0.5	1.2	0.9	0.7	0.6	0.7	0.6
227.4	Benign neoplasm of pineal gland	-	0.0	-	0.0	-	-	-	0.0	-	0.0
230	Carcinoma in situ of digestive organs										
230.0	Lip, oral cavity and pharynx	0.1	0.1	0.1	0.0	0.1	0.1	0.1	0.1	0.1	0.1
230.1	Oesophagus	0.0	0.0	0.0	0.0	0.0	0.0	0.0	0.0	0.0	0.0
230.2	Stomach	0.1	0.1	0.1	0.0	0.1	0.0	0.1	0.0	0.1	0.0
230.3	Colon	0.1	0.0	0.1	0.0	0.1	0.0	0.1	0.0	0.1	0.0
230.4	Rectum	0.1	0.1	0.1	0.0	0.1	0.1	0.1	0.1	0.1	0.1
230.5	Anal canal	-	0.0	-	0.0	-	-	-	0.0	-	0.0
230.6	Anus, unspecified	0.0	0.0	0.0	0.0	-	0.0	0.0	0.0	0.0	0.0
230.7	Other and and unspecified parts of intestine	0.0	-	0.0	-	0.0	-	0.0	-	0.0	-

Table 6 Series MB1 no. 19

Table 6 Crude and directly standardised rates - *continued*

ICD (9th Revision) number	Site description	Crude rate M	Crude rate F	World standard population M	World standard population F	Truncated world standard population M	Truncated world standard population F	European standard population M	European standard population F	England and Wales 1981 standard population M	England and Wales 1981 standard population F
230.8	Liver and biliary system	0.0	0.0	0.0	0.0	-	0.0	0.0	0.0	0.0	0.0
230.9	Other and unspecified digestive organs	-	0.0	-	0.0	-	-	-	0.0	-	0.0
231	Carcinoma in situ of respiratory systems										
231.0	Larynx	0.3	0.1	0.2	0.1	0.3	0.2	0.3	0.1	0.3	0.1
231.1	Trachea	-	-	-	-	-	-	-	-	-	-
231.2	Bronchus and lung	0.1	0.0	0.1	0.0	0.1	0.0	0.1	0.0	0.2	0.0
231.8	Other specified parts	0.0	0.0	0.0	0.0	-	0.0	0.0	0.0	0.0	0.0
231.9	Part unspecified	0.0	0.0	0.0	0.0	0.0	0.0	0.0	0.0	0.0	0.0
232	Carcinoma in situ of skin										
232.0	Skin of lip	0.0	0.0	0.0	0.0	0.0	0.0	0.0	0.0	0.1	0.0
232.1	Eyelid, including canthus	0.1	0.0	0.0	0.0	0.0	0.0	0.1	0.0	0.1	0.0
232.2	Ear and external auricular canal	0.3	0.0	0.2	0.0	0.2	0.0	0.3	0.0	0.3	0.0
232.3	Skin of other and unspecified parts	0.4	0.8	0.3	0.3	0.3	0.4	0.4	0.5	0.5	0.7
232.4	Scalp and skin of neck	0.2	0.1	0.1	0.0	0.2	0.0	0.2	0.0	0.2	0.1
232.5	Skin of trunk, except scrotum	0.3	0.3	0.2	0.1	0.3	0.2	0.3	0.2	0.4	0.2
232.6	Skin of upper limb, including shoulder	0.5	0.3	0.3	0.2	0.5	0.3	0.5	0.2	0.6	0.3
232.7	Skin of lower limb, including hip	0.5	2.2	0.3	1.2	0.4	2.0	0.5	1.7	0.6	2.0
232.8	Other specified sites	0.1	0.0	0.0	0.0	0.1	0.1	0.1	0.0	0.1	0.0
232.9	Site unspecified	0.1	0.3	0.1	0.1	0.1	0.2	0.1	0.2	0.2	0.2
233	Carcinoma in situ of breast and genitourinary system										
233.0	Breast	0.0	3.1	0.0	2.5	0.1	6.4	0.0	3.2	0.0	3.1
233.1	Cervix uteri	-	53.0	-	51.2	-	65.9	-	54.8	-	52.6
233.2	Other and unspecified parts of Uterus	-	0.1	-	0.1	-	0.3	-	0.2	-	0.1
233.3	Other and unspecified female genital organs	-	0.5	-	0.4	-	0.8	-	0.5	-	0.5
233.4	Prostate	0.1	-	0.1	-	0.0	-	0.1	-	0.1	-
233.5	Penis	0.1	-	0.1	-	0.1	-	0.1	-	0.1	-
233.6	Other and unspecified male genital organs	0.0	-	0.0	-	0.0	-	0.0	-	0.0	-
233.7	Bladder	0.8	0.2	0.5	0.1	0.8	0.3	0.8	0.2	0.9	0.2
233.9	Other and unspecified urinary organs	0.0	0.0	0.0	0.0	0.0	0.0	0.0	0.0	0.0	0.0

Table 6 Crude and directly standardised rates - *continued*

ICD (9th Revision) number	Site description	Crude rate M	Crude rate F	World standard population M	World standard population F	Truncated world standard population M	Truncated world standard population F	European standard population M	European standard population F	England and Wales 1981 standard population M	England and Wales 1981 standard population F
234	Carcinoma in situ of other and unspecified sites										
234.0	Eye	0.0	-	0.0	-	0.0	-	0.0	-	0.0	-
234.8	Other specified sites	-	0.0	-	0.0	-	0.0	-	0.0	-	0.0
234.9	Site unspecified	-	0.0	-	0.0	-	0.0	-	0.0	-	0.0
235	Neoplasm of uncertain behaviour of digestive and respiratory systems										
235.0	Major salivary glands	0.1	0.1	0.1	0.1	0.1	0.2	0.1	0.1	0.1	0.1
235.1	Lip, oral cavity and pharynx	0.0	0.0	0.0	0.0	0.0	0.0	0.0	0.0	0.0	0.0
235.2	Stomach, intestines and rectum	0.9	1.2	0.6	0.8	0.7	1.0	0.9	1.0	1.1	1.1
235.3	Liver and biliary passages	0.0	0.0	0.0	0.0	-	0.0	0.0	0.0	0.0	0.0
235.4	Retroperitoneum and peritoneum	0.0	0.0	0.0	0.0	0.0	0.0	0.0	0.0	0.0	0.0
235.5	Other and unspecified digestive organs	0.0	0.0	0.0	0.0	-	0.0	0.0	0.0	0.0	0.0
235.6	Larynx	0.0	-	0.0	-	0.0	-	0.0	-	0.0	-
235.7	Trachea, bronchus and lung	0.1	0.2	0.1	0.1	0.2	0.2	0.1	0.2	0.2	0.2
235.8	Pleura, thymus and mediastinum	0.0	0.0	0.0	0.0	0.1	0.1	0.0	0.0	0.0	0.0
235.9	Other and unspecified respiratory organs	0.0	-	0.0	-	0.0	-	0.0	-	0.0	-
236	Neoplasm of uncertain behaviour of genitourinary organs										
236.0	Uterus	-	1.8	-	1.8	-	1.9	-	1.8	-	1.8
236.1	Placenta	-	0.1	-	0.1	-	0.0	-	0.1	-	0.1
236.2	Ovary	-	0.9	-	0.6	-	1.3	-	0.8	-	0.8
236.3	Other and unspecified female organs	-	0.0	-	0.0	-	0.0	-	0.0	-	0.0
236.4	Testis	0.1	-	0.1	-	0.1	-	0.1	-	0.1	-
236.5	Prostate	0.0	-	0.0	-	0.0	-	0.0	-	0.0	-
236.6	Other and unspecified male genital organs	0.0	-	0.0	-	-	-	0.0	-	0.0	-
236.7	Bladder	0.9	0.4	0.6	0.2	1.1	0.4	0.9	0.3	1.1	0.3
236.9	Other and unspecified urinary organs	0.0	0.0	0.0	0.0	-	-	0.0	0.0	0.0	0.0
237	Neoplasm of uncertain behaviour of endocrine glands and nervous system										
237.0	Pituitary glands and craniopharyngeal duct	0.1	0.2	0.1	0.2	0.1	0.2	0.1	0.2	0.1	0.2
237.1	Pineal gland	0.0	-	0.0	-	0.0	-	0.0	-	0.0	-
237.2	Suprarenal gland	-	0.0	-	0.0	-	0.0	-	0.0	-	0.0
237.3	Paraganglia	0.0	0.1	0.0	0.1	0.0	0.1	0.0	0.1	0.0	0.1
237.4	Other and unspecified endocrine glands	0.0	0.0	0.0	0.0	0.0	0.0	0.0	0.0	0.0	0.0

Table 6 Crude and directly standardised rates - *continued*

ICD (9th Revision) number	Site description	Crude rate M	Crude rate F	World standard population M	World standard population F	Truncated world standard population M	Truncated world standard population F	European standard population M	European standard population F	England and Wales 1981 standard population M	England and Wales 1981 standard population F
237.5	Brain and spinal cord	0.3	0.2	0.2	0.2	0.3	0.2	0.3	0.2	0.3	0.2
237.6	Meninges	-	0.0	-	0.0	-	-	-	0.0	-	0.0
237.7	Neurofibromatosis	0.2	0.1	0.2	0.1	0.2	0.2	0.2	0.1	0.2	0.1
237.9	Other and unspecified parts of nervous system	0.0	0.0	0.0	0.0	0.0	-	0.0	0.0	0.0	0.0
238	Neoplasm of uncertain behaviour of other and unspecified sites and tissues										
238.0	Bone and articular carriage	0.1	0.1	0.1	0.1	0.1	0.1	0.1	0.1	0.1	0.1
238.1	Connective and other soft tissue	0.1	0.1	0.1	0.1	0.1	0.1	0.1	0.1	0.1	0.1
238.2	Skin	0.1	0.1	0.1	0.1	0.1	0.1	0.1	0.1	0.1	0.1
238.3	Breast	-	0.2	-	0.1	-	0.3	-	0.2	-	0.1
238.4	Polycythaemia vera	1.3	0.8	0.8	0.4	1.3	0.5	1.2	0.6	1.4	0.7
238.5	Histiocytic and mast cells	0.0	-	0.0	-	-	-	0.0	-	0.0	-
238.6	Plasma cells	0.1	0.1	0.1	0.0	0.2	0.0	0.1	0.1	0.2	0.1
238.7	Other lymphatic and haematopoietic tissues	0.6	0.7	0.3	0.4	0.3	0.5	0.5	0.5	0.7	0.6
238.8	Other specified sites	0.0	0.0	0.0	0.0	0.1	0.0	0.0	0.0	0.0	0.0
238.9	Site unspecified	0.0	0.0	0.0	0.0	-	-	0.0	0.0	0.0	0.0
239.4	Neoplasm of unspecified nature of bladder	0.2	0.0	0.1	0.0	0.1	0.0	0.2	0.0	0.2	0.0
239.6	Neoplasm of unspecified nature of brain	0.7	0.7	0.5	0.4	0.7	0.4	0.7	0.5	0.7	0.6
239.7	Neoplasm of unspecified nature of other parts of nervous system and pituitary gland only	0.1	0.1	0.1	0.1	0.2	0.1	0.1	0.1	0.1	0.1
630	Hydatidiform mole	-	0.7	-	0.7	-	0.1	-	0.6	-	0.7

Table 7 Series MB1 no. 19

Table 7 Registrations of newly diagnosed cases of cancer: sex and site, 1986

ICD (9th Revision) number	Site description		England and Wales	Northern	Yorkshire	Trent	East Anglian	North West Thames	North East Thames*	South East Thames
	All registrations	M	106,605	7,161	7,911	10,466	4,800	5,764	6,561	7,272
		F	121,186	8,486	9,539	11,472	5,218	6,832	7,285	7,797
140-208	All malignant neoplasms	M	103,495	6,871	7,623	10,156	4,655	5,628	6,423	7,109
		F	102,309	6,549	7,764	9,521	4,355	5,696	6,358	7,035
140	Malignant neoplasm of lip	M	198	18	17	29	23	9	5	15
		F	47	2	3	6	3	3	2	2
141	Malignant neoplasm of tongue	M	328	29	19	29	13	15	15	22
		F	213	24	13	20	9	14	15	14
142	Malignant neoplasm of major salivary glands	M	159	13	8	25	9	13	4	9
		F	154	6	11	13	5	12	4	12
143	Malignant neoplasm of gum	M	75	2	8	6	2	4	9	7
		F	45	2	4	3	1	5	2	7
144	Malignant neoplasm of floor of mouth	M	214	44	19	22	8	6	8	14
		F	58	5	9	5	-	1	1	7
145	Malignant neoplasm of other and unspecified parts of mouth	M	199	25	19	21	6	17	6	12
		F	139	8	13	10	3	6	9	9
146	Malignant neoplasm of oropharynx	M	212	13	9	9	11	9	14	16
		F	101	5	14	4	3	10	4	5
147	Malignant neoplasm of nasopharynx	M	109	8	6	5	5	10	8	12
		F	61	6	3	6	-	7	7	2
148	Malignant neoplasm of hypopharynx	M	207	17	21	20	10	14	11	7
		F	135	12	12	11	8	5	6	12
149	Malignant neoplasm of other and ill-defined sites within the lip, oral cavity and pharynx	M	90	7	12	8	-	5	2	4
		F	43	5	5	1	1	3	4	3
150	Malignant neoplasm of oesophagus	M	2,591	198	145	270	133	131	157	197
		F	1,812	140	130	171	61	94	96	142
151	Malignant neoplasm of stomach	M	6,624	468	503	680	263	336	446	447
		F	4,029	290	313	372	154	198	254	286
152	Malignant neoplasm of small intestine, including duodenum	M	153	4	18	9	5	10	9	8
		F	160	8	10	12	6	6	10	10
153	Malignant neoplasm of colon	M	6,542	440	457	680	310	340	354	427
		F	8,234	516	642	740	383	500	509	614
154	Malignant neoplasm of rectum, rectosigmoid junction and anus	M	5,168	375	427	518	250	221	270	311
		F	4,159	242	344	340	190	250	252	289
155	Malignant neoplasm of liver and intrahepatic bile ducts	M	599	41	62	41	12	42	54	59
		F	389	27	25	36	7	25	28	37
156	Malignant neoplasm of gallbladder and extrahepatic bile ducts	M	477	26	35	61	30	28	17	37
		F	695	52	60	90	30	30	32	35
157	Malignant neoplasm of pancreas	M	2,756	170	180	270	107	171	189	201
		F	2,831	189	210	245	126	164	205	181
158	Malignant neoplasm of retroperitoneum and peritoneum	M	105	9	6	8	8	7	9	4
		F	122	2	8	18	6	4	8	9
159	Malignant neoplasm of other and ill-defined sites within the digestive organs and peritoneum	M	170	24	3	17	3	14	21	15
		F	194	16	8	13	7	11	17	21

* See explanatory note on page 3 regarding apparent decrease of North East Thames figures.

**England and Wales,
regional heath authorities**

South West Thames	Wessex	Oxford	South Western	West Midlands	Mersey	North Western	Wales		Site description	ICD (9th Revision) number
5,864	6,597	4,550	6,836	11,415	5,670	9,337	6,401	M	All registrations	
6,691	7,300	5,293	8,166	12,696	6,477	10,798	7,136	F		
5,744	6,355	4,471	6,588	11,191	5,498	9,058	6,125	M	All malignant neoplasms	140-208
6,125	6,289	4,406	6,921	10,657	5,504	9,091	6,038	F		
6	12	19	12	6	1	5	21	M	Malignant neoplasm of lip	140
6	4	5	2	3	1	1	4	F		
17	12	15	20	44	22	38	18	M	Malignant neoplasm of tongue	141
8	15	14	11	20	17	8	11	F		
9	11	2	7	13	9	14	13	M	Malignant neoplasm of major salivary glands	142
7	9	9	3	19	12	9	23	F		
3	4	3	5	4	4	10	4	M	Malignant neoplasm of gum	143
5	4	2	-	4	-	3	3	F		
2	4	4	7	17	18	28	13	M	Malignant neoplasm of floor of mouth	144
4	3	2	3	6	5	3	4	F		
4	7	6	8	25	16	16	11	M	Malignant neoplasm of other and unspecified parts of mouth	145
12	11	6	8	25	3	8	8	F		
6	4	10	13	24	19	41	14	M	Malignant neoplasm of oropharynx	146
5	3	5	3	11	6	13	10	F		
8	3	2	1	17	4	6	14	M	Malignant neoplasm of nasopharynx	147
3	3	4	2	6	1	7	4	F		
12	8	5	7	27	23	16	9	M	Malignant neoplasm of hypopharynx	148
10	3	3	10	12	5	13	13	F		
8	6	4	5	3	6	10	10	M	Malignant neoplasm of other and ill-defined sites within the lip, oral cavity and pharynx	149
2	1	2	3	3	2	5	3	F		
145	171	55	170	265	118	259	177	M	Malignant neoplasm of oesophagus	150
89	120	62	115	191	110	189	102	F		
318	372	254	334	823	358	603	419	M	Malignant neoplasm of stomach	151
192	188	159	245	456	241	416	265	F		
8	11	10	3	25	13	9	11	M	Malignant neoplasm of small intestine, including duodenum	152
9	5	5	9	30	5	14	21	F		
373	467	319	423	717	354	537	344	M	Malignant neoplasm of colon	153
490	578	358	542	860	382	697	423	F		
215	299	195	308	680	283	425	391	M	Malignant neoplasm of rectum, rectosigmoid junction and anus	154
253	248	162	295	391	240	379	284	F		
21	38	18	33	54	37	46	41	M	Malignant neoplasm of liver and intrahepatic bile ducts	155
20	32	11	29	34	21	35	22	F		
24	15	19	25	59	24	50	27	M	Malignant neoplasm of gallbladder and extrahepatic bile ducts	156
37	39	24	46	86	23	69	42	F		
171	169	112	177	287	133	243	176	M	Malignant neoplasm of pancreas	157
167	187	125	205	275	146	261	145	F		
4	8	4	3	8	7	11	9	M	Malignant neoplasm of retroperitoneum and peritoneum	158
6	10	3	7	7	11	11	12	F		
7	21	1	6	-	2	17	19	M	Malignant neoplasm of other and ill-defined sites within the digestive organs and peritoneum	159
21	18	4	14	-	1	21	22	F		

Table 7 Series MB1 no. 19

Table 7 Registrations in regional health authorities - *continued*

ICD (9th Revision) number	Site description		England and Wales	Northern	Yorkshire	Trent	East Anglian	North West Thames	North East Thames*	South East Thames
160	Malignant neoplasm of nasal cavities, middle ear and accessory sinuses	M F	214 154	9 12	13 3	19 12	16 10	16 12	12 13	19 13
161	Malignant neoplasm of larynx	M F	1,465 319	108 21	105 27	138 34	53 12	100 7	94 19	95 17
162	Malignant neoplasm of trachea, bronchus and lung	M F	24,365 9,991	1,864 774	1,761 777	2,448 889	900 365	1,298 560	1,698 662	1,670 781
163	Malignant neoplasm of pleura	M F	504 97	52 8	33 10	21 8	18 4	27 3	39 10	35 7
164	Malignant neoplasm of thymus, heart and mediastinum	M F	69 51	7 1	4 1	10 4	1 2	5 3	4 5	4 9
165	Malignant neoplasm of other and ill-defined sites within the respiratory system and intrathoracic organs	M F	7 1	- -	- -	- -	1 -	- -	- -	- -
170	Malignant neoplasm of bone and articular cartilage	M F	221 216	13 11	13 9	23 29	11 6	17 11	15 17	23 14
171	Malignant neoplasm of connective and other soft tissue	M F	453 423	40 31	24 24	38 42	24 24	34 24	25 28	28 22
172	Malignant melanoma of skin	M F	989 1,813	58 82	62 138	83 140	44 93	55 85	67 83	67 149
173	Other malignant neoplasm of skin	M F	14,152 12,615	742 751	1,154 1,091	1,282 1,186	777 627	595 511	681 567	1,011 783
174	Malignant neoplasm of female breast	F	22,757	1,257	1,516	2,128	956	1,423	1,592	1,503
175	Malignant neoplasm of male breast	M	155	3	8	16	13	17	11	10
179	Malignant neoplasm of uterus, part unspecified	F	380	26	30	65	5	-	-	-
180	Malignant neoplasm of cervix uteri	F	4,034	280	337	403	135	185	227	240
181	Malignant neoplasm of placenta	F	11	2	1	1	-	1	1	-
182	Malignant neoplasm of body of uterus	F	3,432	190	254	347	173	184	217	266
183	Malignant neoplasm of ovary and other uterine adnexa	F	4,507	280	309	406	210	253	287	305
184	Malignant neoplasm of other and unspecified female genital organs	F	976	65	77	100	52	43	47	58
185	Malignant neoplasm of prostate	M	10,180	535	747	902	543	587	644	727
186	Malignant neoplasm of testis	M	1,022	67	53	95	48	62	60	65
187	Malignant neoplasm of penis and other male genital organs	M	316	17	26	26	12	14	20	15
188	Malignant neoplasm of bladder	M F	6,781 2,810	385 187	483 229	633 234	298 108	417 159	460 185	487 198

* See explanatory note on page 3 regarding apparent decrease of North East Thames figures.

South West Thames	Wessex	Oxford	South Western	West Midlands	Mersey	North Western	Wales		Site description	ICD (9th Revision) number
9	14	12	8	17	12	23	15	M	Malignant neoplasm of nasal cavities, middle ear and accessory sinuses	160
5	13	2	6	18	8	11	16	F		
65	82	54	71	169	77	142	112	M	Malignant neoplasm of larynx	161
20	14	10	16	32	24	37	29	F		
1,294	1,361	943	1,217	2,702	1,454	2,378	1,377	M	Malignant neoplasm of trachea, bronchus and lung	162
600	566	406	510	907	684	980	530	F		
22	64	14	43	32	40	48	16	M	Malignant neoplasm of pleura	163
3	3	5	5	6	10	11	4	F		
8	4	1	3	8	7	1	2	M	Malignant neoplasm of thymus, heart and mediastinum	164
3	4	3	4	4	1	2	5	F		
-	1	-	-	-	-	2	3	M	Malignant neoplasm of other and ill-defined sites within the respiratory system and intrathoracic organs	165
-	-	-	-	-	-	-	1	F		
7	14	8	13	19	3	10	32	M	Malignant neoplasm of bone and articular cartilage	170
24	14	11	6	14	10	13	27	F		
26	37	13	33	53	17	39	22	M	Malignant neoplasm of connective and other soft tissue	171
23	32	14	27	33	16	37	46	F		
59	81	47	94	106	30	76	60	M	Malignant melanoma of skin	172
121	152	100	179	202	66	116	107	F		
850	756	824	1,011	1,638	811	1,203	817	M	Other malignant neoplasm of skin	173
847	631	651	873	1,406	819	1,187	685	F		
1,440	1,536	996	1,609	2,472	1,115	1,849	1,365	F	Malignant neoplasm of female breast	174
16	12	8	9	7	5	10	10	M	Malignant neoplasm of male breast	175
-	46	-	36	38	13	77	44	F	Malignant neoplasm of uterus, part unspecified	179
164	209	140	309	475	246	385	299	F	Malignant neoplasm of cervix uteri	180
	-	1	1	1	-	2	-	F	Malignant neoplasm of placenta	181
229	209	179	245	400	137	217	185	F	Malignant neoplasm of body of uterus	182
296	272	200	277	530	211	409	262	F	Malignant neoplasm of ovary and other uterine adnexa	183
35	73	41	68	104	51	89	73	F	Malignant neoplasm of other and unspecified female genital organs	184
658	768	488	801	1,044	432	758	546	M	Malignant neoplasm of prostate	185
70	75	56	88	105	37	78	63	M	Malignant neoplasm of testis	186
20	19	17	20	38	21	26	25	M	Malignant neoplasm of penis and other male genital organs	187
417	441	291	405	676	358	618	412	M	Malignant neoplasm of bladder	188
147	164	111	171	276	169	311	161	F		

Table 7 Series MB1 no. 19

Table 7 Registrations in regional health authorities - *continued*

ICD (9th Revision) number	Site description		England and Wales	Northern	Yorkshire	Trent	East Anglian	North West Thames	North East Thames*	South East Thames
189	Malignant neoplasm of kidney and other and unspecified urinary organs	M F	1,906 1,185	124 81	153 102	185 120	94 50	105 68	103 69	124 78
190	Malignant neoplasm of eye	M F	186 155	13 8	13 8	21 16	3 9	22 13	15 8	13 16
191	Malignant neoplasm of brain	M F	1,520 1,104	81 66	89 86	141 102	93 65	93 78	76 76	105 72
192	Malignant neoplasm of other and unspecified parts of nervous system	M F	51 53	8 9	3 -	6 3	3 1	6 5	1 2	7 7
193	Malignant neoplasm of thyroid gland	M F	213 521	11 38	9 38	25 59	11 30	12 45	12 27	10 31
194	Malignant neoplasm of other endocrine glands and related structures	M F	65 83	3 2	4 3	4 8	2 8	8 6	8 7	7 8
195	Malignant neoplasm of other and ill-defined sites	M F	148 268	17 39	5 18	31 36	2 13	2 8	3 3	7 3
196	Secondary and unspecified malignant neoplasm of lymph nodes	M F	314 270	40 30	35 23	48 41	17 10	19 13	15 14	13 14
197	Secondary malignant neoplasm of respiratory and digestive systems	M F	1,654 1,710	119 107	158 182	210 183	72 73	117 126	114 108	126 152
198	Secondary malignant neoplasm of other specified sites	M F	808 825	62 58	80 87	116 81	29 17	59 64	46 62	51 68
199	Malignant neoplasm without specification of site	M F	2,316 2,493	173 229	184 190	238 233	76 69	127 110	165 198	134 135
200	Lymphosarcoma and reticulosarcoma	M F	303 231	17 9	38 20	28 21	3 3	9 8	9 14	17 11
201	Hodgkin's disease	M F	693 460	43 41	45 34	71 39	26 28	42 27	56 28	36 20
202	Other malignant neoplasm of lymphoid and histiocytic tissue	M F	2,174 1,924	118 109	115 117	219 180	110 89	154 128	145 140	148 148
203	Multiple myeloma and immunoproliferative neoplasms	M F	1,152 1,018	59 67	84 59	126 79	50 42	50 69	72 69	81 71
204-208	All leukaemias	M F	2,123 1,801	152 121	148 127	225 176	97 63	157 116	145 108	150 139
204	Lymphoid leukaemia	M F	938 710	69 40	63 39	97 73	41 24	78 49	59 41	60 48
205	Myeloid leukaemia	M F	978 904	68 63	67 70	107 93	48 34	61 55	66 49	70 76
206	Monocytic leukaemia	M F	41 51	2 5	3 4	7 6	3 3	1 -	1 1	1 4
207	Other specified leukaemia	M F	22 18	3 3	1 1	5 1	1 -	- 1	1 1	1 1

* See explanatory note on page 3 regarding apparent decrease of North East Thames figures.

South West Thames	Wessex	Oxford	South Western	West Midlands	Mersey	North Western	Wales		Site description	ICD (9th Revision) number
105	133	84	127	201	90	168	110	M	Malignant neoplasm of kidney and other and unspecified urinary organs	189
47	76	47	85	134	48	115	65	F		
19	11	3	11	9	4	17	12	M	Malignant neoplasm of eye	190
12	6	5	10	12	5	17	10	F		
85	107	76	97	162	80	129	106	M	Malignant neoplasm of brain	191
69	69	57	63	97	54	75	75	F		
2	2	1	2	4	2	2	2	M	Malignant neoplasm of other and unspecified parts of nervous system	192
4	2	4	2	5	3	1	5	F		
9	16	12	25	23	11	18	9	M	Malignant neoplasm of thyroid gland	193
29	23	28	37	51	17	38	30	F		
5	3	4	4	2	2	6	3	M	Malignant neoplasm of other endocrine glands and related structures	194
3	6	6	5	4	4	5	8	F		
7	16	1	13	-	6	11	27	M	Malignant neoplasm of other and ill-defined sites	195
9	38	1	22	-	14	22	42	F		
12	19	9	13	25	12	26	11	M	Secondary and unspecified malignant neoplasm of lymph nodes	196
7	13	18	9	17	21	30	10	F		
112	69	92	60	87	117	137	64	M	Secondary malignant neoplasm of respiratory and digestive systems	197
117	75	97	78	87	102	160	63	F		
41	25	39	29	68	61	76	26	M	Secondary malignant neoplasm of other specified sites	198
67	26	42	23	52	50	96	32	F		
83	123	58	182	400	99	138	136	M	Malignant neoplasm without specification of site	199
112	148	58	193	429	120	154	115	F		
13	16	16	57	27	13	28	12	M	Lymphosarcoma and reticulosarcoma	200
6	10	12	42	28	13	26	8	F		
40	41	27	51	62	32	72	49	M	Hodgkin's disease	201
34	18	20	36	39	20	45	31	F		
153	180	82	219	184	92	162	93	M	Other malignant neoplasm of lymphoid and histiocytic tissue	202
143	139	66	158	168	105	138	96	F		
67	73	51	115	136	38	75	75	M	Multiple myeloma and immunoproliferative neoplasms	203
65	85	38	96	87	40	90	61	F		
109	150	83	200	89	84	197	137	M	All leukaemias	204-208
98	136	72	168	90	76	184	127	F		
50	72	35	97	50	31	85	51	M	Lymphoid leukaemia	204
50	56	26	73	37	31	74	49	F		
43	71	42	89	30	46	99	71	M	Myeloid leukaemia	205
38	68	38	72	46	36	98	68	F		
1	3	3	6	3	2	3	2	M	Monocytic leukaemia	206
1	3	1	10	3	3	6	1	F		
4	1	-	1	-	-	3	1	M	Other specified leukaemia	207
-	2	-	3	2	1	1	1	F		

Table 7 Series MB1 no. 19

Table 7 Registrations in regional health authorities - *continued*

ICD (9th Revision) number	Site description		England and Wales	Northern	Yorkshire	Trent	East Anglian	North West Thames	North East Thames*	South East Thames
208	Leukaemia of unspecified cell type	M F	**144** **118**	10 10	14 13	9 3	4 2	17 11	18 16	18 10
223.3	Benign neoplasm of bladder	M F	**28** **14**	1 -	- -	5 2	- 2	- -	- -	- -
225	Benign neoplasm of brain and other parts of nervous system	M F	**288** **558**	26 34	30 50	31 75	7 24	12 40	20 26	15 37
227.3	Benign neoplasm of pituitary gland and craniopharyngeal duct	M F	**163** **152**	10 7	16 11	20 26	12 4	9 4	8 9	9 15
227.4	Benign neoplasm of pineal gland	M F	**-** **1**	- -	- -	- -	- -	- -	- 1	- -
230	Carcinoma in situ of digestive organs	M F	**103** **81**	11 2	5 10	11 8	6 7	3 4	4 3	4 2
231	Carcinoma in situ of respiratory systems	M F	**112** **48**	7 3	13 5	10 2	5 -	5 4	4 3	8 3
232	Carcinoma in situ of skin	M F	**629** **1,048**	33 58	85 134	50 82	23 35	28 53	29 36	36 47
233	Carcinoma in situ of breast and genitourinary system	M F	**261** **14,659**	91 1,398	50 1,388	15 1,569	6 685	7 923	3 786	9 570
233.1	Carcinoma in situ of cervix uteri	F	**13,609**	1,325	1,295	1,491	651	809	688	447
234	Carcinoma in situ of other and unspecified sites	M F	**5** **9**	1 -	- 1	- 1	1 -	- -	- -	- -
235	Neoplasm of uncertain behaviour of digestive and respiratory systems	M F	**310** **419**	22 19	26 37	37 33	18 36	14 39	16 16	24 25
236	Neoplasm of uncertain behaviour of genitourinary organs	M F	**263** **819**	12 351	17 58	31 31	39 22	7 15	8 11	6 6
237	Neoplasm of uncertain behaviour of endocrine glands and nervous system	M F	**157** **165**	9 9	11 17	10 14	10 6	7 9	9 7	12 7
238	Neoplasm of uncertain behaviour of other and unspecified sites and tissues	M F	**546** **525**	38 21	29 31	57 47	14 20	32 29	23 17	21 30
239.4	Neoplasm of unspecified nature of bladder	M F	**48** **8**	8 3	- -	3 -	- 1	3 -	- -	1 -
239.6	Neoplasm of unspecified nature of brain	M F	**164** **174**	19 16	2 5	24 28	3 5	9 14	11 10	15 19
239.7	Neoplasm of unspecified nature of other parts of nervous system and pituitary gland only	M F	**33** **26**	2 3	4 1	6 3	1 1	- 2	3 2	3 1
630	Hydatidiform mole	F	**171**	13	27	30	15	-	-	-

54

Series MB1 no. 19 Table 7

South West Thames	Wessex	Oxford	South Western	West Midlands	Mersey	North Western	Wales		Site description	ICD (9th Revision) number
11	3	3	7	6	5	7	12	M	Leukaemia of unspecified cell type	208
9	7	7	10	2	5	5	8	F		
-	3	-	4	-	1	-	14	M	Benign neoplasm of bladder	223.3
-	-	-	1	-	2	-	7	F		
12	30	15	17	23	7	27	16	M	Benign neoplasm of brain and	225
27	39	25	39	40	20	65	17	F	other parts of nervous system	
-	10	15	23	9	5	12	5	M	Benign neoplasm of pituitary gland	227.3
7	10	13	16	4	4	10	12	F	and craniopharyngeal duct	
-	-	-	-	-	-	-	-	M	Benign neoplasm of pineal gland	227.4
-	-	-	-	-	-	-	-	F		
4	2	8	6	11	2	12	14	M	Carcinoma in situ of digestive	230
2	6	3	6	6	3	7	12	F	organs	
7	6	6	5	6	6	16	8	M	Carcinoma in situ of respiratory	231
6	4	-	2	-	2	10	4	F	systems	
22	27	20	34	83	84	58	17	M	Carcinoma in situ of skin	232
39	45	28	67	151	112	126	35	F		
6	5	7	14	12	14	14	8	M	Carcinoma in situ of breast and	233
413	754	808	895	1,726	646	1,307	791	F	genitourinary system	
291	716	795	839	1,700	593	1,222	747	F	Carcinoma in situ of cervix uteri	233.1
-	-	-	2	1	-	-	-	M	Carcinoma in situ of other and	234
-	-	-	-	-	-	-	7	F	unspecified sites	
21	32	-	26	14	18	24	18	M	Neoplasm of uncertain behaviour of	235
13	34	-	46	27	15	39	40	F	digestive and respiratory systems	
5	13	-	12	15	-	41	57	M	Neoplasm of uncertain behaviour of	236
8	24	3	26	14	140	41	69	F	genitourinary organs	
4	5	-	15	16	5	15	29	M	Neoplasm of uncertain behaviour of	237
8	10	-	14	15	4	17	28	F	endocrine glands and nervous system	
28	58	8	74	26	12	41	85	M	Neoplasm of uncertain behaviour of	238
28	45	7	91	29	16	42	72	F	other and unspecified sites and tissues	
-	29	-	2	-	-	2	-	M	Neoplasm of unspecified nature of	239.4
-	3	-	1	-	-	-	-	F	bladder	
9	18	-	13	8	15	15	3	M	Neoplasm of unspecified nature of	239.6
13	15	-	9	17	7	13	3	F	brain	
2	4	-	1	-	3	2	2	M	Neoplasm of unspecified nature of	239.7
2	2	-	3	-	2	3	1	F	other parts of nervous system and pituitary gland only	
-	20	-	29	10	-	27	-	F	Hydatidiform mole	630

55

Table 8 Series MB1 no. 19

Table 8 Standardised registration ratios: sex and site 1986
(England and Wales = 100)

ICD (9th Revision) number	Site description		Northern	Yorkshire	Trent	East Anglian	North West Thames	North East Thames*	South East Thames	South West Thames
	All registrations	M	**111**	**105**	**106**	**106**	**82**	**83**	**89**	**89**
		F	**115**	**109**	**105**	**108**	**85**	**81**	**83**	**87**
140-208	**All malignant neoplasms**	M	**110**	**104**	**106**	**106**	**83**	**84**	**90**	**90**
		F	**105**	**105**	**104**	**107**	**86**	**84**	**87**	**94**
140	Malignant neoplasm of lip	M	*150*	*121*	158	274	69	*34*	99	49
		F	*72*	*88*	145	159	101	*57*	52	194
141	Malignant neoplasm of tongue	M	*144*	*81*	95	96	68	*62*	90	85
		F	*186*	*85*	105	106	101	*95*	83	58
142	Malignant neoplasm of major salivary glands	M	*136*	*71*	170	134	123	*34*	74	91
		F	*64*	*99*	94	82	118	*35*	99	71
143	Malignant neoplasm of gum	M	*44*	*150*	86	64	80	*162*	124	65
		F	*73*	*123*	75	56	173	*60*	195	172
144	Malignant neoplasm of floor of mouth	M	*330*	*125*	110	92	42	*50*	89	*16*
		F	*140*	*215*	96	..	27	*23*	153	*108*
145	Malignant neoplasm of other and unspecified parts of mouth	M	*205*	*134*	113	73	129	*41*	80	*33*
		F	*94*	*130*	80	54	67	*88*	83	*136*
146	Malignant neoplasm of oropharynx	M	*100*	*60*	45	126	64	*89*	101	*47*
		F	*80*	*193*	44	75	152	*54*	64	*79*
147	Malignant neoplasm of nasopharynx	M	*119*	*77*	49	112	136	*99*	150	*122*
		F	*159*	*68*	108	-	171	*154*	43	*80*
148	Malignant neoplasm of hypopharynx	M	*133*	143	103	*117*	*102*	*72*	*45*	*95*
		F	*145*	123	91	*149*	*58*	*60*	*113*	*116*
149	Malignant neoplasm of other and ill-defined sites within the lip, oral cavity and pharynx	M	*127*	*188*	95	-	84	*30*	59	*146*
		F	*190*	*161*	26	58	107	*126*	89	*73*
150	Malignant neoplasm of oesophagus	M	126	79	112	121	77	82	99	91
		F	129	99	107	84	81	72	97	75
151	Malignant neoplasm of stomach	M	118	107	111	93	78	91	88	77
		F	121	107	105	96	77	85	87	72
152	Malignant neoplasm of small intestine, including duodenum	M	*43*	*166*	*63*	79	98	79	70	85
		F	*82*	*87*	*84*	94	58	85	79	88
153	Malignant neoplasm of colon	M	112	99	112	111	79	73	85	92
		F	104	108	102	117	95	83	92	91
154	Malignant neoplasm of rectum, rectosigmoid junction and anus	M	120	117	108	114	65	71	79	67
		F	96	114	92	115	94	82	86	94
155	Malignant neoplasm of liver and intrahepatic bile ducts	M	112	146	74	48	106	122	130	57
		F	115	89	104	45	100	97	119	79
156	Malignant neoplasm of gallbladder and extrahepatic bile ducts	M	90	104	138	147	90	48	101	81
		F	124	119	147	108	68	62	62	82
157	Malignant neoplasm of pancreas	M	102	92	106	91	95	93	95	100
		F	111	103	98	111	91	98	79	90
158	Malignant neoplasm of retroperitoneum and peritoneum	M	*139*	*80*	81	185	100	*116*	51	*63*
		F	*27*	*91*	164	124	50	*89*	95	*78*
159	Malignant neoplasm of other and ill-defined sites within the digestive organs and peritoneum	M	*235*	*25*	108	41	126	*167*	*114*	*66*
		F	*140*	*57*	77	90	89	*117*	*131*	*162*
160	Malignant neoplasm of nasal cavities, middle ear and accessory sinuses	M	*69*	*85*	95	179	113	*76*	118	*69*
		F	*129*	*27*	88	163	120	*114*	106	*50*

* See explanatory note on page 3 regarding apparent decrease of North East Thames figures.

Series MB1 no. 19 Table 8

England and Wales, regional health authorities

Wessex	Oxford	South Western	West Midlands	Mersey	North Western	Wales		Site description	ICD (9th Revision) number
101	**98**	**90**	**108**	**117**	**114**	**104**	M	**All registrations**	
100	**101**	**98**	**107**	**112**	**111**	**102**	F		
100	**99**	**90**	**109**	**117**	**114**	**102**	M	**All malignant neoplasms**	140-208
101	**102**	**97**	**107**	**113**	**110**	**101**	F		
99	*220*	*85*	*30*	*11*	*33*	*183*	M	Malignant neoplasm of lip	140
137	*266*	*59*	*68*	*45*	*26*	*145*	F		
62	*102*	*89*	*132*	*144*	*149*	*95*	M	Malignant neoplasm of tongue	141
115	*158*	*73*	*98*	*168*	*47*	*89*	F		
113	*28*	*63*	*82*	*124*	*114*	*143*	M	Malignant neoplasm of major salivary glands	142
97	*136*	*28*	*127*	*164*	*73*	*258*	F		
89	*91*	*96*	*53*	*116*	*173*	*92*	M	Malignant neoplasm of gum	143
145	*108*	-	*93*	-	*83*	*114*	F		
32	*42*	*48*	*77*	*179*	*168*	*105*	M	Malignant neoplasm of floor of mouth	144
85	*84*	*74*	*106*	*180*	*64*	*117*	F		
59	*68*	*58*	*124*	*174*	*104*	*96*	M	Malignant neoplasm of other and unspecified parts of mouth	145
131	*103*	*83*	*184*	*45*	*71*	*98*	F		
32	*106*	*90*	*111*	*193*	*249*	*114*	M	Malignant neoplasm of oropharynx	146
49	*116*	*43*	*110*	*124*	*161*	*169*	F		
47	*40*	*14*	*151*	*78*	*71*	*223*	M	Malignant neoplasm of nasopharynx	147
83	*147*	*49*	*98*	*34*	*143*	*114*	F		
65	*55*	*49*	*128*	*240*	*100*	*75*	M	Malignant neoplasm of hypopharynx	148
37	*54*	*105*	*91*	*78*	*119*	*164*	F		
111	*101*	*80*	*33*	*144*	*144*	*191*	M	Malignant neoplasm of other and ill-defined sites within the lip, ral cavity and pharynx	149
38	*111*	*100*	*72*	*97*	*145*	*120*	F		
108	*49*	*92*	*103*	*100*	*130*	*118*	M	Malignant neoplasm of oesophagus	150
107	*85*	*88*	*111*	*129*	*129*	*96*	F		
91	*89*	*70*	*126*	*120*	*119*	*109*	M	Malignant neoplasm of stomach	151
75	*98*	*84*	*121*	*127*	*128*	*113*	F		
120	*147*	*28*	*162*	*184*	*76*	*125*	M	Malignant neoplasm of small intestine, including duodenum	152
51	*76*	*80*	*193*	*66*	*108*	*224*	F		
115	*113*	*90*	*111*	*120*	*107*	*91*	M	Malignant neoplasm of colon	153
114	*107*	*92*	*110*	*98*	*105*	*88*	F		
94	*87*	*84*	*132*	*121*	*107*	*131*	M	Malignant neoplasm of rectum, rectosigmoid junction and anus	154
97	*96*	*100*	*99*	*122*	*113*	*117*	F		
105	*68*	*79*	*90*	*135*	*99*	*118*	M	Malignant neoplasm of liver and intrahepatic bile ducts	155
134	*69*	*105*	*92*	*114*	*112*	*97*	F		
51	*92*	*73*	*125*	*111*	*137*	*98*	M	Malignant neoplasm of gallbladder and extrahepatic bile ducts	156
91	*85*	*93*	*131*	*70*	*123*	*103*	F		
100	*94*	*90*	*105*	*106*	*115*	*110*	M	Malignant neoplasm of pancreas	157
107	*110*	*101*	*103*	*109*	*114*	*87*	F		
129	*85*	*42*	*75*	*143*	*135*	*148*	M	Malignant neoplasm of retroperitoneum and peritoneum	158
136	*58*	*83*	*58*	*188*	*112*	*168*	F		
199	*14*	*49*	-	*26*	*131*	*193*	M	Malignant neoplasm of other and ill-defined sites within the digestive organs and peritoneum	159
148	*51*	*99*	-	*11*	*134*	*195*	F		
08	*126*	*54*	*79*	*122*	*139*	*121*	M	Malignant neoplasm of nasal cavities, middle ear and accessory sinuses	160
138	*31*	*55*	*122*	*109*	*89*	*178*	F		

Table 8 Series MB1 no. 19

Table 8 Standardised registration ratios - *continued*

ICD (9th Revision) number	Site description		Northern	Yorkshire	Trent	East Anglian	North West Thames	North East Thames*	South East Thames	South West Thames
161	Malignant neoplasm of larynx	M	120	101	101	87	103	87	86	73
		F	106	118	118	95	34	81	69	100
162	Malignant neoplasm of trachea, bronchus and lung	M	126	102	108	87	82	94	89	86
		F	126	108	99	92	88	90	99	95
163	Malignant neoplasm of pleura	M	167	92	45	86	81	104	93	72
		F	133	143	92	104	48	140	93	49
164	Malignant neoplasm of thymus, heart and mediastinum	M	165	81	155	36	106	78	79	194
		F	32	27	87	99	88	131	231	94
165	Malignant neoplasm of other and ill-defined sites within the respiratory system and intrathoracic organs	M	-	-	-	338	-	-	-	-
		F	-	-	-	-	-	-	-	-
170	Malignant neoplasm of bone and articular cartilage	M	96	82	111	123	113	92	144	54
		F	83	58	148	70	75	105	86	182
171	Malignant neoplasm of connective and other soft tissue	M	145	74	90	129	111	74	84	95
		F	120	79	110	143	85	89	68	87
172	Malignant melanoma of skin	M	95	88	90	109	81	91	92	99
		F	73	106	85	130	69	61	109	108
173	Other malignant neoplasm of skin	M	87	115	98	130	64	65	94	97
		F	99	120	106	125	63	61	78	104
174	Malignant neoplasm of female breast	F	90	93	103	106	95	94	86	100
175	Malignant neoplasm of male breast	M	32	73	111	199	165	96	85	167
179	Malignant neoplasm of uterus, part unspecified	F	112	110	192	33	-	-	-	-
180	Malignant neoplasm of cervix uteri	F	113	117	109	84	67	75	80	66
181	Malignant neoplasm of placenta	F	300	128	98	-	121	116	-	-
182	Malignant neoplasm of body of uterus	F	89	103	112	127	83	86	100	106
183	Malignant neoplasm of ovary and other uterine adnexa	F	100	95	100	118	86	86	88	105
184	Malignant neoplasm of other and unspecified female genital organs	F	111	109	116	133	68	65	74	55
185	Malignant neoplasm of prostate	M	89	104	96	122	89	86	91	102
186	Malignant neoplasm of testis	M	107	73	99	119	84	77	89	116
187	Malignant neoplasm of penis and other male genital organs	M	90	116	89	89	67	86	62	102
188	Malignant neoplasm of bladder	M	94	101	101	103	94	92	94	99
		F	110	113	94	96	89	89	88	81
189	Malignant neoplasm of kidney and other and unspecified urinary organs	M	106	113	104	118	83	73	87	90
		F	112	119	113	106	89	79	84	63
190	Malignant neoplasm of eye	M	114	98	121	39	175	108	95	170
		F	84	72	115	147	127	69	134	124
191	Malignant neoplasm of brain	M	86	82	99	151	90	67	95	94
		F	96	108	101	149	106	93	87	102

* See explanatory note on page 3 regarding apparent decrease of North East Thames figures.

Wessex	Oxford	South Western	West Midlands	Mersey	North Western	Wales		Site description	ICD (9th Revision) number
93	84	70	114	114	125	131	M	Malignant neoplasm of larynx	161
73	75	72	102	157	144	154	F		
91	90	70	112	131	127	97	M	Malignant neoplasm of trachea, bronchus and lung	162
93	99	73	93	143	121	90	F		
214	63	124	62	171	123	55	M	Malignant neoplasm of pleura	163
51	124	74	63	215	141	70	F		
99	31	66	113	216	19	51	M	Malignant neoplasm of thymus, heart and mediastinum	164
132	133	116	79	41	49	170	F		
232	-	-	-	-	374	747	M	Malignant neoplasm of other and ill-defined sites within the respiratory system and intrathoracic organs	165
-	-	-	-	-	-	1625	F		
108	75	90	83	29	58	254	M	Malignant neoplasm of bone and articular cartilage	170
110	111	42	65	96	75	218	F		
138	62	108	115	81	110	85	M	Malignant neoplasm of connective and other soft tissue	171
127	75	94	79	79	109	189	F		
140	101	144	104	65	98	107	M	Malignant melanoma of skin	172
142	122	148	111	76	80	103	F		
87	133	101	116	126	111	100	M	Other malignant neoplasm of skin	173
82	125	98	116	137	117	93	F		
113	101	103	110	102	102	103	F	Malignant neoplasm of female breast	174
127	117	82	45	71	84	112	M	Malignant neoplasm of male breast	175
199	-	135	103	72	253	198	F	Malignant neoplasm of uterus, part unspecified	179
89	75	116	117	127	120	130	F	Malignant neoplasm of cervix uteri	180
-	172	149	89	-	232	-	F	Malignant neoplasm of placenta	181
101	124	103	118	83	79	92	F	Malignant neoplasm of body of uterus	182
101	103	90	119	97	113	100	F	Malignant neoplasm of ovary and other uterine adnexa	183
121	103	98	113	111	113	129	F	Malignant neoplasm of other and unspecified female genital organs	184
118	113	106	107	96	98	93	M	Malignant neoplasm of prostate	185
129	106	140	98	76	96	113	M	Malignant neoplasm of testis	186
97	123	89	122	147	107	138	M	Malignant neoplasm of penis and other male genital organs	187
106	99	84	101	116	119	105	M	Malignant neoplasm of bladder	188
95	97	85	103	127	137	98	F		
117	99	96	104	102	114	100	M	Malignant neoplasm of kidney and other and unspecified urinary organs	189
106	95	103	116	85	120	94	F		
101	35	88	47	46	117	112	M	Malignant neoplasm of eye	190
65	74	95	78	67	136	111	F		
122	107	97	102	111	108	122	M	Malignant neoplasm of brain	191
106	115	85	87	101	85	117	F		

Table 8 Series MB1 no. 19

Table 8 Standardised registration ratios - *continued*

ICD (9th Revision) number	Site description		Northern	Yorkshire	Trent	East Anglian	North West Thames	North East Thames*	South East Thames	South West Thames
192	Malignant neoplasm of other and unspecified parts of nervous system	M F	254 273	82 -	126 62	146 48	171 138	26 51	191 182	67 126
193	Malignant neoplasm of thyroid gland	M F	84 119	59 102	126 125	126 146	83 127	76 69	63 79	70 90
194	Malignant neoplasm of other endocrine glands and related structures	M F	75 39	86 50	66 106	76 243	178 107	164 113	149 128	131 59
195	Malignant neoplasm of other and ill-defined sites	M F	189 243	48 93	226 153	32 122	20 47	27 15	62 14	77 51
196	Secondary and unspecified malignant neoplasm of lymph nodes	M F	209 180	157 118	164 169	129 93	91 74	65 70	55 67	62 41
197	Secondary malignant neoplasm of respiratory and digestive systems	M F	120 103	135 147	137 121	102 107	108 115	93 85	99 111	109 106
198	Secondary malignant neoplasm of other specified sites	M F	126 115	139 146	154 110	85 52	111 121	77 102	83 104	83 127
199	Malignant neoplasm without specification of site	M F	125 154	112 105	111 106	76 69	84 69	96 107	74 66	57<
68
200	Lymphosarcoma and reticulosarcoma	M F	92 64	176 120	99 101	24 33	45 53	40 82	75 61	71 41
201	Hodgkin's disease	M F	101 146	91 103	110 93	94 154	86 84	108 80	72 59	98 122
202	Other malignant neoplasm of lymphoid and histiocytic tissue	M F	89 93	74 84	108 104	122 116	106 102	90 98	91 98	116 117
203	Multiple myeloma and immunoproliferative neoplasms	M F	85 109	103 80	118 87	102 103	66 106	85 92	91 87	94 99
204-208	All leukaemias	M F	119 112	98 97	115 110	108 88	112 99	92 80	93 97	83 85
204	Lymphoid leukaemia	M F	123 94	94 76	112 116	103 85	126 106	85 77	84 85	87 109
205	Myeloid leukaemia	M F	116 115	97 107	118 115	116 95	94 93	91 73	94 107	71 66
206	Monocytic leukaemia	M F	82 163	104 108	185 132	170 148	37 -	33 26	31 99	39 31
207	Other specified leukaemia	M F	227 279	64 76	245 63	106<>-	- 84	62 74	59 71	297 -
208	Leukaemia of unspecified cell type	M F	116 143	137 152	68<>29	65 42	180 145	169 182	162 104	123 116
223.3	Benign neoplasm of bladder	M F	58 -	- -	191 155	- 365	- -	- -	- -	- -
225	Benign neoplasm of brain and other parts of nervous system	M F	146 98	146 125	115 148	60 109	61 108	93 63	71 87	69 78
227.3	Benign neoplasm of pituitary gland and craniopharyngeal duct	M F	99 74	138 101	131<>186	184 67	80 38	66 79	76 134	- 76
227.4	Benign neoplasm of pineal gland	M F	: -	: -	: -	: -	: -	: 1349	: -	: -

* See explanatory note on page 3 regarding apparent decrease of North East Thames figures.

Wessex	Oxford	South Western	West Midlands	Mersey	North Western	Wales		Site description	ICD (9th Revision) number
68	*40*	*62*	*75*	*82*	*49*	*69*	M	Malignant neoplasm of other and unspecified parts of nervous system	192
66	*158*	*59*	*91*	*116*	*24*	*165*	F		
127	*123*	174	106	*111*	109	74	M	Malignant neoplasm of thyroid gland	193
75	118	107	98	68	92	101	F		
80	*127*	96	*30*	65	*116*	*81*	M	Malignant neoplasm of other endocrine glands and related structures	194
124	*158*	91	*48*	100	75	*167*	F		
178	*15*	*125*	-	*88*	*96*	317	M	Malignant neoplasm of other and ill-defined sites	195
229	9	114	-	*111*	102	269	F		
100	65	*59*	79	*83*	107	*61*	M	Secondary and unspecified malignant neoplasm of lymph nodes	196
80	159	*48*	64	163	138	*63*	F		
68	129	51	53	*157*	108	67	M	Secondary malignant neoplasm of respiratory and digestive systems	197
71	140	64	53	126	116	63	F		
51	111	51	84	165	122	55	M	Secondary malignant neoplasm of other specified sites	198
52	124	40	65	127	144	66	F		
85	58	108	177	96	78	102	M	Malignant neoplasm without specification of site	199
96	58	107	183	102	77	79	F		
88	*117*	274	88	*93*	119	*69*	M	Lymphosarcoma and reticulosarcoma	200
71	*123*	261	125	*118*	140	*59*	F		
102	78	116	86	97	132	127	M	Hodgkin's disease	201
68	90	121	84	90	123	120	F		
139	83	147	83	91	96	74	M	Other malignant neoplasm of ymphoid and histiocytic tissue	202 l
119	81	118	89	114	89	86	F		
103	102	139	119	73	85	113	M	Multiple myeloma and immunoproliferative neoplasms	203
136	92	132	90	83	109	102	F		
115	87	134	42	87	120	113	M	All leukaemias	204-208
124	94	133	52	89	127	122	F		
125	82	148	53	72	117	95	M	Lymphoid leukaemia	204
129	86	147	55	92	129	119	F		
119	96	130	31	131	127		M	Myeloid leukaemia	205
124	99	114	53	84	135	130	F		
117	*167*	*203*	*75*	*109*	*96*	*85*	M	Monocytic leukaemia	206
97	*47*	*281*	*61*	*124*	*145*	*34*	F		
74	-	64	-	-	176	78	M	Other specified leukaemia	207
185	-	245	*114*	*116*	69	97	F		
34	*48*	*68*	*42*	*77*	*63*	*145*	M	Leukaemia of unspecified cell type	208
96	*145*	*119*	*18*	*90*	*52*	*117*	F		
179	-	209	-	77	-	866	M	Benign neoplasm of bladder	223.3
-	-	109	-	294	-	878	F		
179	*113*	89	77	52	120	97	M	Benign neoplasm of brain and other parts of nervous system	225
118	*102*	103	72	74	146	*53*	F		
107	195	217	*53*	65	94	54	M	Benign neoplasm of pituitary gland and craniopharyngeal duct	227.3
113	183	161	*26*	54	83	139	F		
:	:	:	:	:	:	:	M	Benign neoplasm of pineal gland	227.4
-	-	-	-	-	-	-	F		

Table 8 Series MB1 no. 19

Table 8 Standardised registration ratios - *continued*

ICD (9th Revision) number	Site description		Northern	Yorkshire	Trent	East Anglian	North West Thames	North East Thames*	South East Thames	South West Thames
230	Carcinoma in situ of digestive organs	M F	173 40	68 171	114 110	140 217	44 77	53 50	52 31	64 39
231	Carcinoma in situ of respiratory systems	M F	102 100	163 145	96 46	106 -	68 128	48 85	95 82	103 203
232	Carcinoma in situ of skin	M F	87 91	191 177	86 88	86 84	68 79	62 47	75 57	57 58
233	Carcinoma in situ of breast and genitourinary system	M F	571 157	270 134	62 116	55 118	41 85	16 69	46 54	38 47
233.1	Carcinoma in situ of cervix uteri	F	160	134	119	121	80	65	46	36
234	Carcinoma in situ of other and unspecified sites	M F	317 -	- 155	- 123	485 -	- -	- -	- -	- -
235	Neoplasm of uncertain behaviour of digestive and respiratory systems	M F	116 74	118 123	128 87	140 217	67 140	69 51	103 78	111 50
236	Neoplasm of uncertain behaviour of genitourinary organs	M F	75 700	91 99	127 41	356 68	40 26	41 18	30 10	31 16
237	Neoplasm of uncertain behaviour of endocrine glands and nervous system	M F	93 89	98 143	68 93	158 92	65 79	77 57	106 57	43 80
238	Neoplasm of uncertain behaviour of other and unspecified sites and tissues	M F	115 66	75 82	112 100	61 96	88 84	57 44	51 73	83 84
239.4	Neoplasm of unspecified nature of bladder	M F	279 622	- -	68 -	- 316	95 -	- -	27 -	- -
239.6	Neoplasm of unspecified nature of brain	M F	190 153	17 40	157 181	44 72	82 124	90 77	122 137	90 116
239.7	Neoplasm of unspecified nature of other parts of nervous system and pituitary gland only	M F	98 187	170 53	195 127	74 97	- 115	122 103	124 51	101 125
630	Hydatidiform mole	F	125	221	190	224	-	-	-	-

* See explanatory note on page 3 regarding apparent decrease of North East Thames figures.

Wessex	Oxford	South Western	West Midlands	Mersey	North Western	Wales		Site description	ICD (9th Revision) number
33	*176*	*85*	*105*	*42*	*150*	*234*	M	Carcinoma in situ of digestive	230
121	*90*	*105*	*77*	*78*	*107*	*253*	F	organs	
89	*123*	*64*	*53*	*116*	*184*	*122*	M	Carcinoma in situ of respiratory	231
140	-	*61*	-	*86*	*259*	*142*	F	systems	
70	*73*	*76*	*133*	*294*	*120*	*47*	M	Carcinoma in situ of skin	232
70	*65*	*91*	*149*	*225*	*149*	*57*	F		
32	*61*	*77*	*46*	*117*	*69*	*53*	M	Carcinoma in situ of breast and	233
91	*107*	*98*	*115*	*92*	*114*	*99*	F	genitourinary system	
93	*113*	*100*	*122*	*91*	*115*	*101*	F	Carcinoma in situ of cervix uteri	233.1
-	-	*584*	*194*	-	-	-	M	Carcinoma in situ of other and	234
-	-	-	-	-	-	*1361*	F	unspecified sites	
172	-	*123*	*45*	*126*	*100*	*101*	M	Neoplasm of uncertain behaviour of	235
136	-	*162*	*65*	*75*	*116*	*165*	F	digestive and respiratory systems	
82	-	*66*	*57*	-	*202*	*377*	M	Neoplasm of uncertain behaviour of	236
51	*7*	*50*	*17*	*356*	*63*	*151*	F	genitourinary organs	
55	-	*147*	*98*	*67*	*121*	*324*	M	Neoplasm of uncertain behaviour of	237
104	-	*130*	*90*	*50*	*129*	*299*	F	endocrine glands and nervous system	
175	*33*	*194*	*48*	*48*	*97*	*271*	M	Neoplasm of uncertain behaviour of	238
141	*31*	*249*	*57*	*64*	*99*	*237*	F	other and unspecified sites and tissues	
972	-	*58*	-	-	*54*	-	M	Neoplasm of unspecified nature of	239.4
610	-	*176*	-	-	-	-	F	bladder	
183	-	*115*	*48*	*198*	*118*	*32*	M	Neoplasm of unspecified nature of	239.6
141	-	*73*	*102*	*85*	*93*	*30*	F	brain	
206	-	*45*	-	*194*	*78*	*105*	M	Neoplasm of unspecified nature of	239.7
130	-	*172*	-	*160*	*143*	*67*	F	other parts of nervous system and pituitary gland only	
209	-	*279*	*57*	-	*200*	-	F	Hydatidiform mole	630

Table 9 Series MB1 no. 19

Table 9 Directly age standardised (world standard population) rates of newly diagnosed cases of cancer : sex and site 1986

ICD (9th Revision) number	Site description		England and Wales	Northern	Yorkshire	Trent	East Anglian	North West Thames	North East Thames*	South East Thames
	All registrations	M	276.4	309.4	288.8	292.2	292.1	226.6	229.2	244.0
		F	284.8	344.3	319.5	304.4	308.9	240.4	222.4	221.3
140-208	All malignant neoplasms	M	267.6	295.7	277.2	282.8	281.9	220.9	223.9	237.8
		F	219.3	229.5	233.4	230.3	232.6	186.0	180.3	187.2
140	Malignant neoplasm of lip	M	0.5	0.8	0.6	0.9	1.3	0.4	0.2	0.6
		F	0.1	0.0	0.0	0.1	0.1	0.1	0.0	0.0
141	Malignant neoplasm of tongue	M	0.9	1.4	0.7	0.9	1.0	0.7	0.5	0.8
		F	0.4	0.8	0.4	0.4	0.4	0.5	0.3	0.3
142	Malignant neoplasm of major salivary glands	M	0.4	0.6	0.3	0.8	0.6	0.6	0.1	0.3
		F	0.3	0.2	0.3	0.3	0.4	0.5	0.2	0.3
143	Malignant neoplasm of gum	M	0.2	0.1	0.3	0.2	0.1	0.1	0.3	0.2
		F	0.1	0.0	0.1	0.1	0.0	0.2	0.0	0.2
144	Malignant neoplasm of floor of mouth	M	0.6	2.0	0.8	0.7	0.5	0.3	0.4	0.6
		F	0.1	0.1	0.3	0.1	-	0.0	0.0	0.2
145	Malignant neoplasm of other and unspecified parts of mouth	M	0.6	1.2	0.7	0.7	0.4	0.7	0.2	0.4
		F	0.3	0.2	0.3	0.2	0.2	0.2	0.3	0.2
146	Malignant neoplasm of oropharynx	M	0.6	0.6	0.4	0.2	0.7	0.4	0.5	0.6
		F	0.2	0.2	0.5	0.1	0.1	0.4	0.2	0.2
147	Malignant neoplasm of nasopharynx	M	0.3	0.4	0.3	0.2	0.3	0.4	0.3	0.5
		F	0.2	0.2	0.2	0.1	-	0.3	0.4	0.1
148	Malignant neoplasm of hypopharynx	M	0.6	0.8	0.8	0.5	0.7	0.6	0.4	0.2
		F	0.3	0.6	0.3	0.3	0.4	0.2	0.2	0.2
149	Malignant neoplasm of other and ill-defined sites within the lip, oral cavity and pharynx	M	0.3	0.3	0.4	0.2	-	0.2	0.1	0.2
		F	0.1	0.2	0.1	0.0	0.1	0.1	0.1	0.1
150	Malignant neoplasm of oesophagus	M	6.6	8.5	5.1	7.4	8.0	5.1	5.5	6.5
		F	3.0	3.9	3.0	3.3	2.4	2.4	2.2	2.8
151	Malignant neoplasm of stomach	M	16.4	19.1	18.0	17.8	15.1	12.6	14.7	13.9
		F	6.3	7.8	6.7	6.6	5.8	4.9	5.4	5.4
152	Malignant neoplasm of small intestine, including duodenum	M	0.4	0.2	0.9	0.2	0.4	0.4	0.4	0.3
		F	0.3	0.3	0.3	0.3	0.3	0.2	0.3	0.3
153	Malignant neoplasm of colon	M	16.4	18.6	16.0	18.3	18.0	13.1	12.2	13.8
		F	14.5	14.5	14.8	15.1	17.5	14.1	11.8	12.9
154	Malignant neoplasm of rectum, rectosigmoid junction and anus	M	13.2	16.3	15.4	14.1	15.1	8.3	9.1	10.1
		F	7.5	7.5	8.4	6.9	8.2	7.1	5.6	5.9
155	Malignant neoplasm of liver and intrahepatic bile ducts	M	1.6	1.8	2.4	1.1	0.8	1.7	2.1	2.0
		F	0.7	0.8	0.7	0.7	0.5	0.7	0.8	0.7
156	Malignant neoplasm of gallbladder and extrahepatic bile ducts	M	1.2	1.1	1.2	1.7	1.7	1.2	0.6	1.3
		F	1.2	1.5	1.5	1.7	1.2	0.8	0.8	0.8
157	Malignant neoplasm of pancreas	M	7.0	7.2	6.4	7.4	6.6	6.5	6.4	6.8
		F	4.7	5.4	4.9	4.6	5.2	4.2	4.7	3.7
158	Malignant neoplasm of retroperitoneum and peritoneum	M	0.3	0.4	0.2	0.2	0.7	0.3	0.4	0.2
		F	0.3	0.1	0.3	0.5	0.4	0.1	0.3	0.3
159	Malignant neoplasm of other and ill-defined sites within the digestive organs and peritoneum	M	0.4	1.0	0.1	0.5	0.2	0.5	0.6	0.5
		F	0.3	0.5	0.2	0.2	0.2	0.3	0.3	0.3

* See expanatory note on page 3 regarding apparent decrease of North East Thames figures.

Series MB1 no. 19 Table 9

**England and Wales,
regional health authorities**

South West Thames	Wessex	Oxford	South Western	West Midlands	Mersey	North Western	Wales		Site description	ICD (9th Revision) number
242.7	278.4	268.1	252.5	297.5	322.1	316.6	289.0	M	All registrations	
232.7	283.2	283.8	281.2	307.1	317.1	316.6	298.7	F		
237.1	267.0	263.0	242.3	291.3	312.2	306.5	274.5	M	All malignant neoplasms	140-208
202.7	222.4	221.1	214.6	236.3	247.8	241.6	229.8	F		
0.2	0.5	1.2	0.5	0.2	0.1	0.2	0.9	M	Malignant neoplasm of lip	140
0.1	0.1	0.2	0.0	0.1	0.0	0.0	0.1	F		
0.7	0.6	0.9	0.8	1.3	1.3	1.4	0.9	M	Malignant neoplasm of tongue	141
0.2	0.5	0.7	0.3	0.4	0.6	0.2	0.4	F		
0.5	0.4	0.1	0.2	0.4	0.5	0.5	0.7	M	Malignant neoplasm of major	142
0.2	0.2	0.4	0.1	0.5	0.6	0.2	0.9	F	salivary glands	
0.1	0.2	0.2	0.2	0.1	0.2	0.3	0.2	M	Malignant neoplasm of gum	143
0.2	0.1	0.1	-	0.1	-	0.1	0.1	F		
0.1	0.2	0.3	0.3	0.5	1.1	1.2	0.6	M	Malignant neoplasm of floor of	144
0.1	0.1	0.1	0.1	0.1	0.2	0.1	0.2	F	mouth	
0.2	0.4	0.4	0.3	0.7	1.1	0.5	0.5	M	Malignant neoplasm of other and	145
0.3	0.5	0.3	0.3	0.6	0.2	0.3	0.4	F	unspecified parts of mouth	
0.3	0.2	0.6	0.5	0.7	1.2	1.6	0.8	M	Malignant neoplasm of oropharynx	146
0.2	0.1	0.3	0.1	0.3	0.2	0.4	0.4	F		
0.3	0.2	0.1	0.0	0.5	0.3	0.3	0.7	M	Malignant neoplasm of nasopharynx	147
0.1	0.1	0.2	0.0	0.1	0.0	0.3	0.2	F		
0.5	0.4	0.3	0.3	0.7	1.5	0.5	0.4	M	Malignant neoplasm of hypopharynx	148
0.3	0.1	0.1	0.3	0.3	0.2	0.3	0.4	F		
0.3	0.3	0.2	0.2	0.1	0.3	0.4	0.6	M	Malignant neoplasm of other and	149
0.1	0.1	0.1	0.0	0.1	0.1	0.1	0.1	F	ill-defined sites within the lip, oral cavity and pharynx	
6.2	7.0	3.4	5.8	6.7	6.8	8.8	7.8	M	Malignant neoplasm of oesophagus	150
2.2	3.2	2.6	2.5	3.7	3.8	3.8	2.6	F		
13.2	14.6	14.5	11.4	20.6	20.4	19.5	17.8	M	Malignant neoplasm of stomach	151
4.3	4.6	6.1	5.3	7.5	8.5	7.7	7.1	F		
0.4	0.6	0.7	0.1	0.7	0.8	0.3	0.5	M	Malignant neoplasm of small	152
0.3	0.2	0.2	0.3	0.6	0.1	0.3	0.7	F	intestine, including duodenum	
14.5	18.9	18.6	14.7	18.3	19.7	17.2	15.1	M	Malignant neoplasm of colon	153
13.7	17.2	15.8	13.1	15.7	14.4	15.0	12.8	F		
8.7	12.5	10.7	10.9	17.5	15.9	14.3	17.4	M	Malignant neoplasm of rectum,	154
7.4	7.7	7.0	7.5	7.7	8.7	8.6	9.5	F	rectosigmoid junction and anus	
1.1	1.8	1.1	1.3	1.4	2.1	1.6	1.9	M	Malignant neoplasm of liver and	155
0.7	0.9	0.4	0.7	0.8	0.8	0.9	0.7	F	intrahepatic bile ducts	
0.9	0.6	1.2	0.8	1.5	1.4	1.7	1.2	M	Malignant neoplasm of gallbladder	156
0.9	1.1	1.1	1.1	1.5	0.7	1.4	1.1	F	and extrahepatic bile ducts	
7.1	7.0	6.5	6.3	7.5	7.4	8.0	7.8	M	Malignant neoplasm of pancreas	157
4.1	4.6	5.1	4.7	4.8	5.0	5.6	4.4	F		
0.2	0.4	0.3	0.1	0.2	0.4	0.3	0.4	M	Malignant neoplasm of	158
0.4	0.3	0.1	0.3	0.2	0.6	0.3	0.5	F	retroperitoneum and peritoneum	
0.2	0.8	0.1	0.2	-	0.1	0.5	0.8	M	Malignant neoplasm of other and	159
0.4	0.4	0.2	0.3	-	0.0	0.4	0.5	F	ill-defined sites within the digestive organs and peritoneum	

65

Table 9 Series MB1 no. 19

ICD (9th Revision) number	Site description		England and Wales	Northern	Yorkshire	Trent	East Anglian	North West Thames	North East Thames*	South East Thames
				Regional health authority of residence						
160	Malignant neoplasm of nasal cavities, middle ear and accessory sinuses	M	**0.6**	0.4	0.5	0.6	1.0	0.6	0.5	0.7
		F	**0.3**	0.4	0.1	0.2	0.5	0.3	0.4	0.4
161	Malignant neoplasm of larynx	M	**4.0**	4.9	4.1	4.1	3.5	4.1	3.2	3.3
		F	**0.7**	0.8	1.0	0.9	0.6	0.2	0.6	0.5
162	Malignant neoplasm of trachea, bronchus and lung	M	**61.1**	77.8	63.0	65.7	52.6	49.1	57.6	53.7
		F	**20.1**	26.2	21.9	20.7	18.1	16.5	16.7	19.5
163	Malignant neoplasm of pleura	M	**1.4**	2.3	1.4	0.7	1.4	1.1	1.5	1.2
		F	**0.2**	0.3	0.3	0.2	0.3	0.0	0.3	0.2
164	Malignant neoplasm of thymus, heart and mediastinum	M	**0.2**	0.4	0.2	0.4	0.1	0.2	0.2	0.1
		F	**0.1**	0.0	0.0	0.1	0.2	0.1	0.2	0.4
165	Malignant neoplasm of other and ill-defined sites within the respiratory system and intrathoracic organs	M	**0.0**	-	-	-	0.0	-	-	-
		F	**0.0**	-	-	-	-	-	-	-
170	Malignant neoplasm of bone and articular cartilage	M	**0.8**	0.7	0.6	0.9	0.8	0.8	0.7	1.3
		F	**0.7**	0.5	0.4	1.3	0.6	0.8	0.9	0.6
171	Malignant neoplasm of connective and other soft tissue	M	**1.4**	2.1	1.0	1.4	1.7	1.7	1.2	1.2
		F	**1.2**	1.2	0.9	1.4	1.5	1.1	0.9	0.6
172	Malignant melanoma of skin	M	**3.1**	3.0	2.8	2.7	3.6	2.5	2.8	2.9
		F	**5.2**	3.6	5.5	4.4	6.7	3.5	3.0	5.9
173	Other malignant neoplasm of skin	M	**36.8**	31.5	41.8	36.0	46.8	23.4	23.7	33.9
		F	**23.8**	22.6	29.1	24.2	30.2	15.0	14.3	18.1
174	Malignant neoplasm of female breast	F	**56.9**	52.3	55.0	59.2	59.6	52.7	52.6	47.4
175	Malignant neoplasm of male breast	M	**0.4**	0.1	0.3	0.5	0.8	0.7	0.4	0.3
179	Malignant neoplasm of uterus, part unspecified	F	**0.8**	0.8	0.9	1.6	0.2	-	-	-
180	Malignant neoplasm of cervix uteri	F	**12.0**	13.0	14.7	13.2	9.7	7.8	8.7	9.3
181	Malignant neoplasm of placenta	F	**0.0**	0.1	0.1	0.0	-	0.1	0.0	-
182	Malignant neoplasm of body of uterus	F	**7.9**	7.7	8.0	9.4	9.3	6.4	6.5	7.5
183	Malignant neoplasm of ovary and other uterine adnexa	F	**11.0**	11.3	11.1	11.0	13.2	9.2	8.8	9.1
184	Malignant neoplasm of other and unspecified female genital organs	F	**1.7**	1.9	2.0	2.0	1.9	1.3	1.0	1.2
185	Malignant neoplasm of prostate	M	**23.0**	20.5	24.2	22.4	27.5	20.4	20.1	20.6
186	Malignant neoplasm of testis	M	**3.8**	4.2	2.8	3.8	4.5	3.2	3.1	3.3
187	Malignant neoplasm of penis and other male genital organs	M	**0.8**	0.7	0.9	0.7	0.7	0.5	0.8	0.6
188	Malignant neoplasm of bladder	M	**17.1**	16.1	17.4	17.2	18.1	15.8	15.4	16.0
		F	**5.1**	5.5	6.1	5.0	4.8	4.6	3.9	4.4
189	Malignant neoplasm of kidney and other and unspecified urinary organs	M	**5.3**	5.6	5.9	5.4	6.0	4.3	3.9	4.7
		F	**2.7**	3.0	3.5	3.1	2.9	2.5	2.2	2.4

* See explanatory note on page 3 regarding apparent decrease of North East Thames figures

Series MB1 no. 19 Table 9

South West Thames	Wessex	Oxford	South Western	West Midlands	Mersey	North Western	Wales		Site description	ICD (9th Revision) number
0.5	*0.6*	*0.7*	*0.4*	*0.5*	*0.8*	*0.9*	*0.7*	M	Malignant neoplasm of nasal cavities, middle ear and accessory sinuses	160
0.2	*0.5*	*0.1*	*0.2*	*0.4*	*0.3*	*0.2*	*0.6*	F		
2.9	3.5	3.3	2.6	4.7	4.8	5.0	5.2	M	Malignant neoplasm of larynx	161
0.7	*0.4*	*0.5*	*0.5*	*0.8*	1.1	1.1	1.2	F		
51.5	54.7	54.1	42.6	68.4	80.4	78.2	59.7	M	Malignant neoplasm of trachea, bronchus and lung	162
17.3	18.7	19.1	13.5	19.1	30.6	25.8	18.6	F		
1.0	2.9	*1.0*	1.8	*0.9*	2.3	1.7	*0.7*	M	Malignant neoplasm of pleura	163
0.1	*0.1*	*0.3*	*0.2*	*0.1*	*0.5*	*0.2*	*0.2*	F		
0.4	*0.2*	*0.1*	*0.2*	*0.3*	*0.4*	*0.0*	*0.1*	M	Malignant neoplasm of thymus, heart and mediastinum	164
0.1	*0.3*	*0.2*	*0.1*	*0.1*	*0.0*	*0.0*	*0.2*	F		
-	*0.0*	-	-	-	-	*0.1*	*0.1*	M	Malignant neoplasm of other and ill-defined sites within the respiratory system and intrathoracic organs	165
-	-	-	-	-	-	-	*0.0*	F		
0.4	*0.9*	*0.6*	*0.9*	*0.7*	*0.2*	*0.5*	1.7	M	Malignant neoplasm of bone and articular cartilage	170
1.3	*0.6*	*0.6*	*0.3*	*0.3*	*0.5*	*0.5*	1.3	F		
1.2	2.0	*0.9*	1.3	1.6	*1.0*	1.6	1.1	M	Malignant neoplasm of connective and other soft tissue	171
1.3	1.2	*0.8*	1.2	1.0	*0.9*	1.6	2.0	F		
3.0	4.5	3.1	4.6	3.3	2.1	3.1	3.2	M	Malignant melanoma of skin	172
5.7	7.4	6.0	7.8	5.9	3.8	4.3	5.2	F		
35.0	31.8	49.4	38.2	43.0	46.2	41.0	37.7	M	Other malignant neoplasm of skin	173
23.9	19.6	30.1	25.5	27.7	31.9	27.4	22.8	F		
56.7	63.8	57.8	58.2	61.6	60.2	58.9	59.6	F	Malignant neoplasm of female breast	174
0.7	*0.5*	*0.5*	*0.3*	*0.2*	*0.3*	*0.3*	*0.5*	M	Malignant neoplasm of male breast	175
-	1.4	-	*0.9*	*0.8*	*0.5*	2.2	1.8	F	Malignant neoplasm of uterus, part unspecified	179
7.7	10.9	9.0	13.9	14.3	15.5	14.2	15.9	F	Malignant neoplasm of cervix uteri	180
-	-	*0.1*	*0.1*	*0.0*	-	*0.1*	-	F	Malignant neoplasm of placenta	181
8.3	8.1	9.8	8.1	9.6	6.7	6.4	7.4	F	Malignant neoplasm of body of uterus	182
11.6	10.5	11.8	9.8	13.6	11.2	12.2	11.2	F	Malignant neoplasm of ovary and other uterine adnexa	183
0.7	2.1	1.6	1.6	1.9	1.8	1.8	2.6	F	Malignant neoplasm of other and unspecified female genital organs	184
23.3	27.3	25.5	24.6	24.7	22.0	22.9	20.9	M	Malignant neoplasm of prostate	185
4.5	4.9	3.9	5.5	3.9	2.9	3.7	4.1	M	Malignant neoplasm of testis	186
0.8	*0.8*	*1.1*	*0.7*	1.0	1.2	*0.9*	1.2	M	Malignant neoplasm of penis and other male genital organs	187
16.7	17.8	17.0	14.4	17.2	19.5	20.9	17.6	M	Malignant neoplasm of bladder	188
3.7	4.7	4.7	4.4	**5.3**	6.5	7.2	5.3	F		
4.6	6.1	5.5	5.3	5.6	5.5	6.0	5.4	M	Malignant neoplasm of kidney and other and unspecified urinary organs	189
1.6	2.7	2.6	2.3	3.0	2.1	2.9	2.7	F		

Table 9 Series MB1 no. 19

ICD (9th Revision) number	Site description		England and Wales	Regional health authority of residence						
				Northern	Yorkshire	Trent	East Anglian	North West Thames	North East Thames*	South East Thames
190	Malignant neoplasm of eye	M	0.6	0.7	0.5	0.7	0.3	1.2	0.7	0.6
		F	0.4	0.4	0.3	0.5	0.6	0.5	0.3	0.6
191	Malignant neoplasm of brain	M	5.1	4.6	4.1	5.1	6.9	4.5	3.3	4.8
		F	3.3	3.5	3.5	3.5	4.9	3.5	3.0	2.8
192	Malignant neoplasm of other and unspecified parts of nervous system	M	0.2	0.6	0.2	0.3	0.3	0.4	0.0	0.3
		F	0.2	0.6	-	0.1	0.0	0.4	0.1	0.4
193	Malignant neoplasm of thyroid gland	M	0.6	0.6	0.4	0.8	0.8	0.6	0.5	0.3
		F	1.5	1.6	1.6	1.8	2.1	1.8	1.0	1.2
194	Malignant neoplasm of other endocrine glands and related structures	M	0.3	0.2	0.2	0.2	0.1	0.5	0.3	0.4
		F	0.3	0.2	0.1	0.4	0.6	0.4	0.4	0.4
195	Malignant neoplasm of other and ill-defined sites	M	0.4	0.7	0.2	1.0	0.1	0.1	0.1	0.3
		F	0.5	1.0	0.5	0.7	0.6	0.3	0.1	0.1
196	Secondary and unspecified malignant neoplasm of lymph nodes	M	0.8	1.8	1.3	1.4	1.1	0.8	0.5	0.6
		F	0.6	1.1	0.8	1.1	0.6	0.4	0.4	0.4
197	Secondary malignant neoplasm of respiratory and digestive systems	M	4.1	5.2	5.5	5.7	4.3	4.5	4.1	4.1
		F	3.0	3.3	4.6	3.8	2.9	3.4	2.6	3.6
198	Secondary malignant neoplasm of other specified sites	M	2.1	2.6	3.0	3.5	1.8	2.4	1.5	1.7
		F	1.6	1.9	2.7	2.0	1.0	1.9	1.7	1.7
199	Malignant neoplasm without specification of site	M	5.7	7.0	6.2	6.1	4.2	4.9	5.5	4.4
		F	4.0	6.3	4.4	4.3	3.0	2.5	4.4	2.6
200	Lymphosarcoma and reticulosarcoma	M	0.9	0.7	1.5	0.9	0.2	0.4	0.3	0.7
		F	0.5	0.4	0.5	0.5	0.2	0.2	0.4	0.3
201	Hodgkin's disease	M	2.5	2.6	2.3	2.8	2.4	2.2	2.9	1.9
		F	1.5	2.4	1.7	1.5	2.3	1.2	1.0	0.9
202	Other malignant neoplasm of lymphoid and histiocytic tissue	M	6.3	5.6	4.7	6.9	7.8	6.5	5.6	5.7
		F	4.2	4.0	3.3	4.4	5.1	4.1	4.5	4.3
203	Multiple myeloma and immunoproliferative neoplasms	M	2.9	2.5	3.1	3.5	3.0	1.9	2.4	2.7
		F	1.8	2.0	1.5	1.5	1.5	1.9	1.7	1.7
204-208	All leukaemias	M	6.3	7.9	5.9	7.5	6.8	7.8	6.0	5.5
		F	4.2	4.5	4.1	4.7	3.3	4.2	3.9	4.0
204	Lymphoid leukaemia	M	3.0	4.0	2.6	3.6	2.9	4.2	2.7	2.4
		F	1.8	1.7	1.5	2.1	1.5	1.9	1.9	1.6
205	Myeloid leukaemia	M	2.8	3.3	2.6	3.4	3.4	2.7	2.6	2.5
		F	2.0	2.2	2.0	2.3	1.5	2.0	1.5	2.0
206	Monocytic leukaemia	M	0.1	0.1	0.1	0.2	0.2	0.0	0.0	0.0
		F	0.1	0.2	0.1	0.2	0.2	-	0.0	0.1
207	Other specified leukaemia	M	0.1	0.1	0.0	0.1	0.1	-	0.0	0.0
		F	0.1	0.2	0.1	0.0	-	0.0	0.1	0.0
208	Leukaemia of unspecified cell type	M	0.4	0.4	0.5	0.2	0.2	0.9	0.6	0.6
		F	0.2	0.3	0.4	0.1	0.0	0.3	0.5	0.2
223.3	Benign neoplasm of bladder	M	0.1	0.1	-	0.1	-	-	-	-
		F	0.0	-	-	0.1	0.1	-	-	-

* See expanatory note on page 3 regarding apparent decrease of North East Thames figures

South West Thames	Wessex	Oxford	South Western	West Midlands	Mersey	North Western	Wales		Site description	ICD (9th Revision) number
1.0	0.6	0.2	0.5	0.3	0.2	0.9	0.7	M	Malignant neoplasm of eye	190
0.6	0.6	0.3	0.4	0.3	0.3	0.5	0.4	F		
4.9	6.2	5.5	4.8	5.4	6.0	5.5	5.9	M	Malignant neoplasm of brain	191
3.3	3.5	3.5	2.8	3.1	3.1	3.1	4.1	F		
0.1	0.1	0.1	0.2	0.2	0.2	0.1	0.2	M	Malignant neoplasm of other and unspecified parts of nervous system	192
0.3	0.1	0.3	0.1	0.2	0.3	0.1	0.3	F		
0.4	0.7	0.8	1.0	0.7	0.7	0.7	0.5	M	Malignant neoplasm of thyroid gland	193
1.4	1.2	1.9	1.4	1.4	1.0	1.2	1.5	F		
0.3	0.3	0.5	0.3	0.1	0.1	0.3	0.1	M	Malignant neoplasm of other endocrine glands and related structures	194
0.1	0.2	0.4	0.2	0.1	0.3	0.2	0.5	F		
0.3	0.6	0.1	0.5	-	0.3	0.4	1.5	M	Malignant neoplasm of other and ill-defined sites	195
0.2	1.0	0.0	0.5	-	0.7	0.4	1.5	F		
0.5	0.8	0.4	0.5	0.6	0.7	0.8	0.6	M	Secondary and unspecified malignant neoplasm of lymph nodes	196
0.2	0.5	0.7	0.2	0.4	0.9	0.8	0.4	F		
4.3	2.8	5.3	2.1	2.2	6.4	4.4	2.8	M	Secondary malignant neoplasm of respiratory and digestive systems	197
2.9	2.0	4.2	2.0	1.5	4.0	3.6	1.9	F		
1.8	1.1	2.5	1.0	1.8	3.3	2.5	1.1	M	Secondary malignant neoplasm of other specified sites	198
1.8	0.8	1.5	0.7	1.0	2.1	2.4	1.3	F		
3.4	4.8	3.2	6.2	10.1	5.7	4.3	5.6	M	Malignant neoplasm without specification of site	199
2.5	3.7	2.3	4.1	7.7	3.8	2.9	3.2	F		
0.6	0.9	1.1	2.0	0.8	0.9	1.2	0.6	M	Lymphosarcoma and reticulosarcoma	200
0.2	0.4	0.6	1.5	0.6	0.6	0.6	0.4	F		
2.5	2.6	2.0	3.2	2.2	2.4	3.2	3.1	M	Hodgkin's disease	201
1.9	1.1	1.4	1.7	1.3	1.3	1.7	1.9	F		
7.5	8.9	5.2	9.4	5.3	5.7	5.9	4.8	M	Other malignant neoplasm of lymphoid and histiocytic tissue	202
5.1	5.2	3.2	4.8	3.8	5.1	3.8	3.6	F		
2.6	2.9	2.9	4.2	3.6	2.1	2.6	3.2	M	Multiple myeloma and immunoproliferative neoplasms	203
1.8	2.3	1.6	2.3	1.6	1.7	1.9	2.1	F		
4.6	7.8	5.5	8.4	2.6	5.4	7.6	6.7	M	All leukaemias	204-208
3.4	4.7	3.3	6.2	2.4	3.8	5.1	5.0	F		
2.1	4.0	2.5	4.4	1.5	2.1	3.6	2.6	M	Lymphoid leukaemia	204
1.5	1.7	1.3	2.7	1.1	1.9	2.0	1.9	F		
1.8	3.5	2.7	3.5	0.9	2.9	3.4	3.4	M	Myeloid leukaemia	205
1.5	2.4	1.8	2.8	1.1	1.6	2.7	2.8	F		
0.1	0.1	0.2	0.2	0.1	0.1	0.2	0.1	M	Monocytic leukaemia	206
0.0	0.1	0.0	0.3	0.1	0.1	0.2	0.0	F		
0.2	0.0	-	0.0	-	-	0.1	0.0	M	Other specified leukaemia	207
-	0.3	-	0.1	0.0	0.0	0.0	0.0	F		
0.5	0.1	0.1	0.2	0.1	0.3	0.2	0.6	M	Leukaemia of unspecified cell type	208
0.4	0.2	0.2	0.2	0.0	0.2	0.1	0.2	F		
-	0.2	-	0.1	-	0.1	-	0.7	M	Benign neoplasm of bladder	223.3
-	-	-	0.1	-	0.2	-	0.4	F		

Table 9 Series MB1 no. 19

ICD (9th Revision) number	Site description		England and Wales	Regional health authority of residence						
				Northern	Yorkshire	Trent	East Anglian	North West Thames	North East Thames*	South East Thames
225	Benign neoplasm of brain and other parts of nervous system	M F	0.9 1.5	1.5 1.6	1.4 1.8	1.0 2.4	0.4 1.5	0.5 1.6	0.8 0.8	0.7 1.4
227.3	Benign neoplasm of pituitary gland and craniopharyngeal duct	M F	0.5 0.5	0.5 0.3	0.7 0.5	0.7 0.9	0.9 0.2	0.4 0.2	0.4 0.4	0.5 0.7
227.4	Benign neoplasm of pineal gland	M F	- 0.0	- -	- -	- -	- -	- -	- 0.1	- -
230	Carcinoma in situ of digestive organs	M F	0.3 0.2	0.5 0.0	0.2 0.3	0.3 0.2	0.4 0.3	0.1 0.1	0.1 0.1	0.2 0.0
231	Carcinoma in situ of respiratory systems	M F	0.3 0.1	0.3 0.2	0.5 0.2	0.3 0.1	0.3 -	0.2 0.2	0.2 0.1	0.3 0.1
232	Carcinoma in situ of skin	M F	1.6 2.1	1.5 1.9	3.0 3.5	1.4 1.7	1.5 2.0	1.1 1.7	1.0 1.0	1.2 1.2
233	Carcinoma in situ of breast and genitourinary system	M F	0.7 54.4	4.2 85.2	1.8 72.5	0.4 63.4	0.3 64.2	0.3 46.4	0.1 37.5	0.3 28.2
233.1	Carcinoma in situ of cervix uteri	F	51.2	82.1	68.6	60.9	61.7	41.2	33.6	23.2
234	Carcinoma in situ of other and unspecified sites	M F	0.0 0.0	0.0 -	- 0.0	- 0.0	0.1 -	- -	- -	- -
235	Neoplasm of uncertain behaviour of digestive and respiratory systems	M F	0.9 1.1	1.1 0.9	1.1 1.4	1.0 0.8	1.4 2.9	0.6 1.5	0.6 0.6	0.7 0.8
236	Neoplasm of uncertain behaviour of genitourinary organs	M F	0.7 2.8	0.4 21.7	0.8 2.5	1.0 1.0	2.7 1.3	0.3 0.6	0.3 0.4	0.2 0.2
237	Neoplasm of uncertain behaviour of endocrine glands and nervous system	M F	0.6 0.6	0.5 0.5	0.7 0.6	0.3 0.6	1.0 0.6	0.4 0.6	0.4 0.3	0.6 0.4
238	Neoplasm of uncertain behaviour of other and unspecified sites and tissues	M F	1.5 1.2	1.7 0.8	1.2 1.0	1.7 1.1	0.8 1.1	1.1 1.0	0.7 0.5	0.7 0.7
239.4	Neoplasm of unspecified nature of bladder	M F	0.1 0.0	0.3 0.0	- -	0.1 -	- 0.1	0.1 -	- -	0.0 -
239.6	Neoplasm of unspecified nature of brain	M F	0.5 0.4	0.9 0.6	0.1 0.2	0.8 0.6	0.2 0.2	0.4 0.4	0.4 0.3	0.7 0.4
239.7	Neoplasm of unspecified nature of other parts of nervous system and pituitary gland only	M F	0.1 0.1	0.2 0.2	0.2 0.0	0.2 0.1	0.1 0.1	- 0.1	0.2 0.1	0.1 0.0
630	Hydatidiform mole	F	0.7	0.9	1.5	1.3	1.6	-	-	-

* See expanatory note on page 3 regarding apparent decrease of North East Thames figures

South West Thames	Wessex	Oxford	South Western	West Midlands	Mersey	North Western	Wales		Site description	ICD (9th Revision) number
0.6	1.6	1.0	0.8	0.7	0.4	1.1	0.9	M	Benign neoplasm of brain and	225
1.0	1.7	1.5	1.6	1.1	1.2	2.5	0.8	F	other parts of nervous system	
-	0.6	1.1	1.2	0.3	0.3	0.5	0.3	M	Benign neoplasm of pituitary gland	227.3
0.4	0.5	0.9	0.8	0.1	0.2	0.4	0.8	F	and craniopharyngeal duct	
-	-	-	-	-	-	-	-	M	Benign neoplasm of pineal gland	227.4
-	-	-	-	-	-	-	-	F		
0.2	0.1	0.5	0.2	0.3	0.1	0.4	0.7	M	Carcinoma in situ of digestive	230
0.1	0.1	0.1	0.1	0.1	0.1	0.2	0.4	F	organs	
0.3	0.2	0.3	0.2	0.1	0.3	0.6	0.3	M	Carcinoma in situ of respiratory	231
0.2	0.2	-	0.1	-	0.1	0.3	0.2	F	systems	
1.0	1.2	1.2	1.2	2.1	4.5	2.0	0.8	M	Carcinoma in situ of skin	232
1.2	1.4	1.1	1.9	3.1	4.7	3.0	1.2	F		
0.2	0.2	0.4	0.4	0.3	0.8	0.4	0.5	M	Carcinoma in situ of breast and	233
24.2	49.8	58.6	52.8	63.4	50.0	62.2	54.1	F	genitourinary system	
18.3	47.7	57.8	50.3	62.6	46.5	58.7	51.7	F	Carcinoma in situ of cervix uteri	233.1
-	-	-	0.1	0.0	-	-	-	M	Carcinoma in situ of other and	234
-	-	-	-	-	-	-	0.4	F	unspecified sites	
1.2	1.5	-	1.2	0.4	1.1	0.8	1.0	M	Neoplasm of uncertain behaviour of	235
0.5	1.4	-	1.7	0.9	0.7	1.2	1.5	F	digestive and respiratory systems	
0.2	0.6	-	0.4	0.4	-	1.6	2.8	M	Neoplasm of uncertain behaviour of	236
0.4	1.4	0.2	1.4	0.3	10.7	1.3	3.8	F	genitourinary organs	
0.3	0.3	-	0.8	0.5	0.4	0.7	1.8	M	Neoplasm of uncertain behaviour of	237
0.4	0.5	-	0.8	0.4	0.3	0.8	1.6	F	endocrine glands and nervous system	
1.2	2.6	0.5	2.9	0.7	0.7	1.4	4.7	M	Neoplasm of uncertain behaviour of	238
1.1	1.5	0.3	3.0	0.6	0.7	1.2	3.4	F	other and unspecified sites and tissues	
-	1.2	-	0.1	-	-	0.1	-	M	Neoplasm of unspecified nature of	239.4
-	0.1	-	0.0	-	-	-	-	F	bladder	
0.5	0.9	-	0.4	0.2	1.0	0.6	0.2	M	Neoplasm of unspecified nature of	239.6
0.6	0.6	-	0.3	0.3	0.2	0.3	0.1	F	brain	
0.1	0.2	-	0.1	-	0.2	0.1	0.1	M	Neoplasm of unspecified nature of	239.7
0.1	0.1	-	0.2	-	0.1	0.1	0.1	F	other parts of nervous system and pituitary gland only	
-	1.4	-	1.9	0.4	-	1.4	-	F	Hydatidiform mole	630

Appendix A Series MB1 no. 19

Appendix A Estimated resident population: sex and age as at 30 June 1986

(Figures in thousands)

Area		All ages	Under 1	1-4	5-9	10-14	15-19	20-24	25-29	30-34	35-39
England and Wales	M	**24,403.5**	**336.1**	**1,296.1**	**1,553.3**	**1,651.9**	**2,004.5**	**2,130.4**	**1,877.0**	**1,683.0**	**1,851.2**
	F	**25,671.9**	**318.8**	**1,232.2**	**1,471.3**	**1,561.6**	**1,906.7**	**2,072.2**	**1,847.0**	**1,658.3**	**1,848.7**
England	M	23,034.4	317.1	1,223.4	1,464.4	1,556.1	1,891.6	2,013.1	1,777.8	1,593.8	1,750.8
	F	24,220.0	301.0	1,162.7	1,387.7	1,471.5	1,798.2	1,955.8	1,750.3	1,571.2	1,748.0
Wales	M	1,369.1	18.9	72.7	88.9	95.8	113.0	117.3	99.2	89.1	100.4
	F	1,451.9	17.7	69.5	83.7	90.1	108.5	116.4	96.8	87.0	100.7
Regional health authorities											
Northern	M	1,500.1	20.7	79.8	96.9	103.7	119.2	127.5	114.6	103.6	112.4
	F	1,580.2	19.5	76.0	91.6	98.1	117.1	126.1	112.7	100.3	110.3
Yorkshire	M	1,752.8	24.6	94.1	113.8	122.9	145.9	151.9	133.2	120.3	131.6
	F	1,848.6	23.2	90.3	108.3	116.1	140.7	148.4	130.2	117.2	130.1
Trent	M	2,279.1	30.3	118.3	143.9	156.2	185.1	198.4	174.8	157.1	173.8
	F	2,354.7	28.5	111.4	135.9	147.7	177.4	191.6	170.8	152.1	170.5
East Anglia	M	976.5	12.8	52.2	63.5	65.9	80.1	86.0	71.9	65.3	73.4
	F	1,015.1	12.0	50.1	60.2	62.7	73.4	79.3	72.5	68.2	74.3
North West Thames	M	1,702.6	24.4	91.9	106.0	107.4	133.1	156.0	141.1	125.1	134.4
	F	1,785.5	23.3	87.4	101.3	102.6	130.4	155.3	141.9	126.4	136.6
North East Thames	M	1,824.8	26.5	99.8	114.3	118.0	140.1	163.8	147.1	131.1	140.9
	F	1,936.1	25.4	95.4	109.1	111.1	138.2	165.7	149.1	131.0	142.8
South East Thames	M	1,739.4	23.9	90.5	106.6	112.2	140.3	150.8	134.3	120.8	131.0
	F	1,879.2	23.0	86.1	101.3	106.6	136.1	149.3	133.3	119.1	131.8
South West Thames	M	1,429.0	18.6	72.1	86.0	90.2	115.9	117.6	109.9	101.2	113.0
	F	1,535.5	17.7	69.0	82.1	86.0	107.0	116.3	107.6	99.8	114.3
Wessex	M	1,402.3	18.0	71.4	87.0	92.6	123.6	127.2	109.0	93.4	102.6
	F	1,474.1	17.1	67.2	81.3	87.1	108.8	114.0	102.5	93.2	104.8
OxFord	M	1,230.2	17.1	68.7	82.9	85.2	112.6	115.7	99.1	87.9	97.2
	F	1,246.1	16.3	64.8	77.7	80.3	99.6	108.0	97.6	88.8	97.3
South Western	M	1,534.6	19.6	76.1	93.9	100.8	127.5	129.3	111.1	100.8	113.0
	F	1,642.9	18.4	72.4	89.1	96.0	118.9	124.4	110.7	101.7	115.2
West Midlands	M	2,555.7	35.6	137.7	165.7	180.5	212.7	218.8	193.9	173.8	193.8
	F	2,625.5	33.9	129.8	156.5	169.3	202.1	212.1	187.5	166.9	189.8
Mersey	M	1,169.2	16.7	63.8	77.0	84.2	97.2	101.0	89.2	79.7	86.7
	F	1,245.0	15.8	60.7	72.7	79.1	94.8	100.0	88.9	78.4	87.0
North Western	M	1,938.3	28.2	107.1	126.8	136.2	158.2	169.0	148.6	133.6	146.9
	F	2,051.6	26.9	102.1	120.6	128.8	153.7	165.4	144.9	128.2	143.2
England and Wales, metropolitan counties, predominantly urban and predominantly rural aggregates*											
Metropolitan Counties	M	8,718.1	128.8	478.2	551.3	580.1	693.2	792.4	699.2	617.8	659.3
	F	9,223.0	122.5	454.8	523.5	547.9	684.1	785.5	695.4	604.3	653.1
Urban areas	M	11,573.2	156.6	610.2	741.6	791.2	955.4	995.9	875.5	790.5	880.2
	F	12,189.9	148.6	581.9	703.3	750.1	906.6	966.0	858.6	779.6	881.2
Rural areas	M	4,112.2	50.6	207.7	260.3	280.6	356.0	342.0	302.3	274.6	311.7
	F	4,259.0	47.6	195.5	244.5	263.6	316.0	320.7	293.1	274.4	314.4
Wales											
Urban areas	M	981.8	14.0	53.2	64.3	68.9	79.7	84.1	71.5	64.2	72.4
	F	1,045.1	13.2	51.0	60.5	65.1	77.7	84.0	70.4	63.0	72.7
Rural areas	M	387.3	4.9	19.6	24.6	26.9	33.3	33.2	27.7	24.9	28.0
	F	406.8	4.6	18.6	23.2	25.0	30.8	32.4	26.4	24.1	28.0
Standard regions											
North											
Metropolitan Counties	M	549.7	7.8	29.3	34.7	37.0	43.1	48.3	43.2	38.5	40.3
	F	585.7	7.4	27.9	32.9	35.1	43.0	47.4	42.3	36.8	39.4
Urban areas	M	814.2	11.4	44.1	53.9	57.7	64.7	68.9	61.9	56.1	61.9
	F	850.4	10.6	42.2	51.1	54.8	63.6	68.3	60.8	54.9	61.0
Rural areas	M	136.1	1.5	6.4	8.3	9.0	11.3	10.3	9.5	9.0	10.2
	F	144.0	1.5	5.9	7.6	8.2	10.5	10.3	9.6	8.6	9.9

* For definition of metropolitan counties, predominantly urban and predominantly rural, see pages 5 and 7.

Series MB1 no. 19 Appendix A

England and Wales, England, Wales,
regional health authorities, standard regions,
metropolitan counties, predominantly urban
and predominantly rural aggregates.

40-44	45-49	50-54	55-59	60-64	65-69	70-74	75-79	80-84	85+		Area
1,593.2	**1,394.2**	**1,334.0**	**1,328.9**	**1,299.4**	**1,071.5**	**897.2**	**625.9**	**325.9**	**150.0**	M	**England and Wales**
1,570.1	**1,382.0**	**1,332.7**	**1,374.0**	**1,415.1**	**1,279.3**	**1,210.1**	**1,014.0**	**688.6**	**489.0**	F	
1,505.7	1,316.1	1,259.0	1,253.1	1,221.7	1,006.5	844.8	590.5	307.5	141.6	M	England
1,483.3	1,304.9	1,256.7	1,295.2	1,329.3	1,200.6	1,138.7	954.6	648.5	461.7	F	
87.5	78.2	75.0	75.8	77.7	65.0	52.3	35.5	18.4	8.4	M	Wales
86.8	77.1	76.0	78.9	85.8	78.7	71.4	59.4	40.1	27.3	F	
											Regional health authorities
96.8	86.6	84.9	86.1	84.4	67.3	53.7	35.9	17.9	7.9	M	Northern
94.6	85.9	85.4	89.5	91.9	81.0	73.8	60.3	39.9	26.2	F	
113.4	99.8	95.4	95.5	93.1	76.5	63.6	43.9	22.8	10.3	M	Yorkshire
110.6	98.7	96.0	99.2	101.1	91.4	87.3	73.7	50.5	35.5	F	
150.8	131.4	125.6	126.0	123.6	101.0	83.2	57.3	29.3	12.9	M	Trent
145.8	128.7	123.6	127.0	130.3	116.8	108.5	89.1	59.1	39.9	F	
63.2	54.6	51.5	50.8	51.0	45.1	39.2	28.1	15.0	7.1	M	East Anglia
61.6	52.9	50.8	53.0	55.8	51.2	49.2	40.8	27.2	19.7	F	
114.4	99.3	94.3	92.3	86.7	68.2	57.3	40.3	20.7	9.6	M	North West Thames
113.2	98.2	92.8	92.0	90.0	79.8	75.5	63.5	43.4	31.8	F	
118.9	102.9	99.2	99.7	96.7	78.5	65.9	46.2	24.2	11.0	M	North East Thames
118.7	102.4	98.6	101.2	102.6	92.3	88.3	74.6	51.5	38.1	F	
111.3	97.0	92.8	93.4	93.9	80.3	70.0	50.2	27.1	13.0	M	South East Thames
111.7	98.2	95.5	100.2	105.8	98.7	96.6	83.5	58.3	44.3	F	
96.6	83.4	79.4	78.4	75.6	62.6	55.0	40.5	21.8	11.0	M	South West Thames
96.9	84.8	81.3	83.2	85.0	77.6	76.6	66.7	47.3	36.1	F	
87.0	76.3	73.6	73.1	73.5	64.2	56.1	40.6	22.1	11.0	M	Wessex
89.2	78.7	75.8	79.4	83.4	77.3	74.7	63.4	43.6	32.4	F	
82.2	69.7	64.2	61.0	57.0	45.9	37.8	26.1	13.5	6.3	M	Oxford
80.7	67.8	61.9	60.9	59.5	52.1	47.7	39.3	26.4	19.4	F	
98.1	86.3	83.2	83.7	85.1	74.4	65.4	47.3	26.0	12.9	M	South Western
98.3	87.3	85.3	90.1	96.3	89.6	87.0	73.8	50.8	37.9	F	
170.6	150.2	143.7	142.7	137.2	109.9	88.2	59.3	29.3	12.2	M	West Midlands
164.2	145.2	138.9	142.3	145.3	128.2	116.7	94.3	61.6	40.7	F	
75.6	67.9	66.2	65.7	61.9	49.4	40.2	27.3	13.5	6.0	M	Mersey
75.3	68.0	66.7	68.5	69.0	61.3	57.3	47.4	31.9	22.1	F	
126.8	110.6	104.9	104.7	101.9	83.3	69.2	47.5	24.1	10.3	M	North Western
122.4	108.0	104.2	108.5	113.2	103.3	99.6	84.2	56.9	37.5	F	
											England and Wales
561.2	492.4	475.5	478.7	463.4	371.1	307.9	212.4	107.9	47.2	M	Metropolitan Counties
550.0	487.1	473.0	488.8	500.4	449.6	426.8	359.5	244.5	172.2	F	
760.7	664.6	633.5	630.6	617.6	512.8	427.8	298.4	156.7	73.3	M	Urban areas
751.1	659.7	636.3	655.2	676.0	612.0	577.4	483.5	328.6	234.3	F	
271.3	237.2	225.0	219.6	218.4	187.6	161.5	115.1	61.3	29.5	M	Rural areas
269.0	235.1	223.5	230.1	238.7	217.8	205.9	171.0	115.6	82.6	F	
											Wales
63.0	56.2	53.8	54.6	55.6	46.1	36.8	24.8	12.8	5.8	M	Urban areas
62.4	55.3	54.4	56.6	61.5	56.4	51.0	42.5	28.4	19.1	F	
24.5	22.0	21.2	21.2	22.1	18.9	15.5	10.6	5.5	2.6	M	Rural areas
24.4	21.7	21.5	22.3	24.2	22.3	20.5	17.0	11.7	8.2	F	
											Standard regions
											North
34.3	31.0	31.1	32.1	31.6	25.1	19.9	13.0	6.5	2.8	M	Metropolitan Counties
33.6	31.1	31.7	33.7	34.9	31.0	28.3	23.3	15.5	10.3	F	
53.5	47.7	46.2	46.3	44.8	35.4	27.9	18.5	9.1	4.1	M	Urban areas
52.4	47.0	45.9	47.4	48.3	41.9	37.6	30.3	19.8	12.7	F	
8.9	7.9	7.7	7.7	8.0	6.8	5.9	4.3	2.3	1.1	M	Rural areas
8.6	7.9	7.8	8.4	8.7	8.1	7.9	6.8	4.6	3.1	F	

Appendix A Series MB1 no. 19

Appendix A Estimated resident population - *continued*

Area		All ages	Under 1	1-4	5-9	10-14	15-19	20-24	25-29	30-34	35-39
Yorkshire and Humberside											
Metropolitan Counties	M	1,634.7	23.2	88.6	106.3	114.7	133.2	143.5	125.8	113.0	123.1
	F	1,716.2	22.0	84.1	100.6	108.1	130.2	140.9	123.8	109.5	120.6
Urban areas	M	453.6	6.5	23.5	28.4	31.5	38.2	39.4	33.9	30.1	32.8
	F	486.1	5.9	22.8	27.1	29.8	38.2	38.6	33.0	29.4	32.7
Rural areas	M	300.3	3.5	14.6	18.6	20.4	26.0	25.2	23.0	20.7	23.2
	F	308.3	3.4	13.9	17.6	19.2	22.6	23.6	21.7	20.3	23.4
North West											
Metropolitan Counties	M	1,962.1	29.2	109.2	128.6	139.1	163.4	175.9	152.8	135.3	145.5
	F	2,085.0	27.5	104.2	122.1	131.0	159.2	171.6	150.2	130.8	143.5
Urban areas	M	1,074.8	14.7	58.2	70.9	76.5	86.3	88.0	79.7	73.3	82.7
	F	1,135.9	14.3	55.2	66.9	72.1	83.5	87.7	78.5	71.1	81.2
Rural areas	M	56.3	0.7	2.7	3.3	3.8	4.6	4.9	4.2	3.7	4.2
	F	60.3	0.7	2.6	3.2	3.7	4.6	4.7	4.0	3.5	4.3
East Midlands											
Urban areas	M	1,552.3	21.2	83.2	100.4	107.2	126.2	135.4	120.0	108.3	119.5
	F	1,605.3	20.2	79.0	95.4	101.9	121.2	133.0	118.1	105.2	117.5
Rural areas	M	377.3	4.5	18.4	23.9	26.2	31.6	30.8	26.9	25.3	29.8
	F	385.0	4.2	17.3	22.2	24.6	28.5	28.4	26.5	25.4	29.7
West Midlands											
Metropolitan Counties	M	1,298.8	19.3	72.4	84.8	91.7	107.5	115.4	100.0	86.7	93.8
	F	1,333.6	18.5	68.0	79.6	85.6	104.0	111.1	95.7	81.9	90.6
Urban areas	M	940.9	12.7	50.3	61.7	67.2	76.8	78.4	71.4	66.5	75.9
	F	967.2	12.1	47.6	58.5	63.3	73.1	77.6	70.3	64.9	75.1
Rural areas	M	316.0	3.7	14.9	19.1	21.6	28.4	25.1	22.5	20.5	24.1
	F	324.7	3.4	14.2	18.4	20.4	25.0	23.4	21.5	20.1	24.1
East Anglia											
Urban areas	M	348.3	5.1	19.5	23.3	23.6	30.1	35.7	27.2	23.5	25.6
	F	367.2	4.7	18.9	22.3	22.6	28.3	32.6	27.8	25.2	26.6
Rural areas	M	628.1	7.7	32.7	40.2	42.3	49.9	50.3	44.7	41.8	47.7
	F	647.9	7.2	31.2	37.9	40.1	45.1	46.6	44.7	42.9	47.7
South East											
Metropolitan Counties	M	3,272.7	49.3	178.7	196.9	197.7	245.9	309.3	277.4	244.3	256.6
	F	3,502.5	47.2	170.5	188.2	188.2	247.7	314.5	283.4	245.3	259.0
Urban areas	M	4,090.3	53.8	212.8	259.1	273.8	344.3	351.1	311.8	281.4	312.8
	F	4,312.1	51.5	203.2	246.4	259.7	317.2	333.0	301.6	277.9	316.4
Rural areas	M	1,033.6	13.5	55.0	68.2	71.9	95.2	91.3	80.8	71.9	80.5
	F	1,053.5	12.7	51.0	63.1	66.6	81.4	85.0	77.9	72.3	81.5
South West											
Urban areas	M	1,317.0	17.1	65.4	79.7	84.7	109.1	114.9	98.1	87.0	96.6
	F	1,420.6	16.1	62.2	75.1	80.7	103.7	111.3	98.1	87.9	97.9
Rural areas	M	877.2	10.7	43.3	54.1	58.6	75.6	71.0	63.0	56.8	63.9
	F	928.4	10.1	40.8	51.2	55.7	67.6	66.2	60.8	57.1	65.8

40-44	45-49	50-54	55-59	60-64	65-69	70-74	75-79	80-84	85+		Area
											Yorkshire and HuMberside
106.0	92.8	89.0	89.6	87.6	71.2	58.4	39.8	20.3	8.7	M	Metropolitan Counties
102.5	91.4	88.7	91.6	94.3	84.7	80.0	66.9	45.4	31.0	F	
28.7	25.8	24.9	25.2	24.9	20.6	17.4	12.2	6.4	3.1	M	Urban areas
28.2	25.8	25.6	26.8	27.5	25.4	24.5	20.7	14.1	10.0	F	
20.1	17.7	16.7	16.2	15.8	13.2	11.3	8.0	4.2	1.9	M	Rural areas
20.0	17.6	16.7	16.9	17.0	15.2	14.1	11.7	7.8	5.5	F	
											North West
125.3	111.0	107.0	107.1	102.9	82.8	68.0	46.1	23.0	9.9	M	Metropolitan Counties
122.6	109.5	107.1	111.4	115.2	104.1	98.8	82.7	55.7	37.8	F	
72.2	63.2	60.0	59.3	57.2	46.8	39.0	26.9	13.8	6.0	M	Urban areas
70.3	62.1	59.7	61.5	62.9	56.8	54.6	46.0	31.1	20.4	F	
3.8	3.5	3.3	3.3	3.1	2.5	2.1	1.4	0.7	0.4	M	Rural areas
3.9	3.5	3.4	3.5	3.4	3.1	2.8	2.4	1.7	1.2	F	
											East Midlands
102.9	88.7	84.2	84.4	82.2	67.0	55.0	38.0	19.5	8.8	M	Urban areas
99.2	86.4	82.6	84.8	86.1	76.9	71.5	59.2	39.5	27.5	F	
26.1	22.5	21.0	20.4	20.2	17.3	14.5	10.1	5.3	2.5	M	Rural areas
25.4	21.9	20.3	20.7	21.4	19.4	18.1	14.6	9.7	6.6	F	
											West Midlands
82.4	74.1	72.8	73.8	71.6	56.9	45.1	30.0	14.6	5.8	M	Metropolitan Counties
79.0	71.6	70.1	73.2	75.7	66.7	60.6	49.0	31.9	20.8	F	
66.6	57.0	52.8	51.4	48.6	38.5	30.6	20.3	10.0	4.1	M	Urban areas
63.9	54.8	51.3	51.3	51.3	44.8	40.4	32.3	20.9	13.7	F	
21.6	19.1	18.1	17.5	17.1	14.5	12.6	9.0	4.7	2.2	M	Rural areas
21.3	18.8	17.5	17.8	18.3	16.7	15.8	13.0	8.8	6.2	F	
											East Anglia
21.5	18.5	17.6	17.6	17.2	14.6	12.3	8.7	4.7	2.2	M	Urban areas
21.7	18.2	17.5	18.1	18.9	17.2	16.5	13.8	9.3	6.8	F	
41.7	36.1	33.9	33.2	33.8	30.5	26.9	19.4	10.4	4.9	M	Rural areas
40.0	34.7	33.3	35.0	36.9	34.1	32.7	27.0	17.9	12.9	F	
											South East
213.1	183.6	175.7	176.0	169.7	135.1	116.5	83.4	43.6	20.0	M	Metropolitan Counties
212.2	183.5	175.4	179.0	180.2	163.1	159.1	137.7	95.9	72.2	F	
269.3	234.4	223.8	220.8	214.5	179.8	152.6	108.3	57.8	28.1	M	Urban areas
269.7	236.1	226.7	231.8	237.0	215.1	205.4	173.6	120.2	89.7	F	
69.0	59.6	55.4	52.4	49.7	40.9	34.5	24.5	13.0	6.3	M	Rural areas
69.1	59.0	54.1	53.7	53.8	47.7	44.4	36.9	24.9	18.3	F	
											South West
83.1	73.1	70.1	71.1	72.6	63.9	56.1	40.6	22.4	11.2	M	Urban areas
83.4	73.9	72.5	76.9	82.5	77.5	76.0	65.2	45.3	34.4	F	
55.5	48.9	47.7	47.7	48.5	42.9	38.2	27.8	15.2	7.6	M	Rural areas
56.3	50.1	48.8	51.7	54.9	51.2	49.6	41.7	28.3	20.6	F	

Appendix B Series MB1 no. 19

APPENDIX B Registrations of newly diagnosed cases of cancer: area of registration and area of residence, 1986

Registry area of registration		Total (all registrations)	Regional health authority of residence							
			Northern	Yorkshire	Trent	East Anglian	North West Thames	North East Thames*	South East Thames	South West Thames
Total (all registrations)	M	106,830	7,161	7,911	10,466	4,800	5,764	6,561	7,272	5,864
	F	121,446	8,486	9,539	11,472	5,218	6,832	7,285	7,797	6,691
Northern	M	7,166	7,160	5	-	-	-	-	-	-
	F	8,484	8,482	2	-	-	-	-	-	-
Yorkshire	M	7,920	-	7,904	10	-	-	-	-	-
	F	9,553	2	9,535	11	-	-	-	-	-
Trent	M	10,369	-	-	10,368	-	-	-	-	-
	F	11,355	-	-	11,355	-	-	-	-	-
East Anglia	M	5,056	-	-	73	4,798	56	81	-	-
	F	5,534	-	1	88	5,217	85	78	-	-
Thames	M	25,202	-	-	-	-	5,608	6,479	7,271	5,840
	F	28,243	-	-	-	-	6,591	7,201	7,793	6,657
Wessex	M	6,406	-	-	-	-	-	-	-	1
	F	7,093	-	-	-	-	-	-	-	-
Oxford	M	4,906	1	1	14	2	100	1	1	23
	F	5,731	1	-	14	1	156	6	4	34
South Western	M	6,833	-	-	-	-	-	-	-	-
	F	8,160	-	-	-	-	-	-	-	-
West Midlands	M	11,378	-	-	1	-	-	-	-	-
	F	12,651	-	-	2	-	-	-	-	-
Mersey	M	5,888	-	1	-	-	-	-	-	-
	F	6,749	-	1	1	-	-	-	-	-
North Western	M	9,311	-	-	-	-	-	-	-	-
	F	10,762	1	-	1	-	-	-	-	-
Wales	M	6,395	-	-	-	-	-	-	-	-
	F	7,131	-	-	-	-	-	-	-	-

* See explanatory note on page 3 regarding apparent decrease of North East Thames figures.

Series MB1 no. 19 Appendix B

**England and Wales,
regional health authorities**

Wessex	Oxford	South Western	West Midlands	Mersey	North Western	Wales	Resident outside England and Wales		Registry area of registration
6,597	4,550	6,836	11,415	5,670	9,337	6,401	225	M	Total
7,300	5,293	8,166	12,696	6,477	10,798	7,136	260	F	(all registrations)
-	-	-	-	-	1	-	-	M	Northern
-	-	-	-	-	-	-	-	F	
-	-	-	-	-	2	-	4	M	Yorkshire
-	-	-	-	-	2	-	3	F	
-	1	-	-	-	-	-	-	M	Trent
-	-	-	-	-	-	-	-	F	
-	19	-	-	-	-	-	29	M	East Anglia
-	28	-	-	-	-	-	37	F	
-	1	1	1	-	-	1	-	M	Thames
-	-	1	-	-	-	-	-	F	
6,405	-	-	-	-	-	-	-	M	Wessex
7,091	1	1	-	-	-	-	-	F	
184	4,526	22	19	-	1	2	9	M	Oxford
203	5,263	20	24	-	1	-	4	F	
8	1	6,812	10	-	1	1	-	M	South Western
6	1	8,144	7	-	-	1	1	F	
-	1	1	11,375	-	-	-	-	M	West Midlands
-	-	-	12,647	-	-	2	-	F	
-	-	-	9	5,667	24	5	182	M	Mersey
-	-	-	16	6,473	38	6	214	F	
-	-	-	-	3	9,308	-	-	M	North Western
-	-	-	-	3	10,757	-	-	F	
-	1	-	1	-	-	6,392	1	M	Wales
-	-	-	2	1	-	7,127	1	F	

Appendix C Cancer incidence to mortality ratios: sex and site, 1986

ICD (9th Revision) number	Site description		England and Wales	Northern	Yorkshire	Trent	East Anglian	North West Thames	North East Thames*	South East Thames
140-208	**All malignant neoplasms**	M	**1.42**	**1.37**	**1.44**	**1.51**	**1.60**	**1.29**	**1.19**	**1.27**
		F	**1.55**	**1.53**	**1.65**	**1.68**	**1.75**	**1.34**	**1.30**	**1.35**
140	Malignant neoplasm of lip	M	**8.65**	18.00	5.67	29.00	:	9.00	:	7.50
		F	**4.27**	2.00	3.00	6.00	:	:	2.00	2.00
141	Malignant neoplasm of tongue	M	**1.57**	1.38	1.19	1.93	1.86	1.50	1.15	1.29
		F	**1.47**	2.67	2.60	1.67	3.00	1.17	2.14	1.00
142	Malignant neoplasm of major salivary glands	M	**1.73**	2.60	1.33	3.57	4.50	1.86	1.00	3.00
		F	**2.80**	3.00	2.75	2.60	2.50	6.00	2.00	2.00
143	Malignant neoplasm of gum	M	**1.56**	:	2.67	0.75	:	1.33	2.25	3.50
		F	**1.00**	0.50	2.00	1.00	:	1.00	0.40	1.75
144	Malignant neoplasm of floor of mouth	M	**2.64**	5.50	2.37	3.14	2.00	1.50	1.14	3.50
		F	**1.49**	1.67	4.50	1.00	-	0.33	0.50	2.33
145	Malignant neoplasm of other and unspecified parts of mouth	M	**2.01**	3.57	2.37	1.91	6.00	1.31	1.00	2.40
		F	**2.24**	2.00	6.50	3.33	3.00	1.00	1.12	3.00
146	Malignant neoplasm of oropharynx	M	**1.61**	1.62	0.90	1.00	5.50	1.29	1.40	2.67
		F	**1.70**	1.25	1.56	4.00	3.00	2.50	1.67	0.71
147	Malignant neoplasm of nasopharynx	M	**1.16**	2.00	2.00	0.62	1.25	1.00	0.67	2.00
		F	**1.03**	1.20	1.00	1.00	-	1.75	2.33	0.67
148	Malignant neoplasm of hypopharynx	M	**1.66**	2.12	1.75	1.18	2.50	1.56	2.20	1.40
		F	**1.26**	1.20	1.33	1.57	2.00	2.50	0.86	1.50
149	Malignant neoplasm of other and ill-defined sites within the lip oral cavity and pharynx	M	**0.96**	0.64	1.20	1.14	-	1.00	0.67	1.33
		F	**0.63**	0.83	0.45	1.00	0.50	0.50	0.50	0.37
150	Malignant neoplasm of oesophagus	M	**0.99**	1.06	0.84	1.10	1.00	0.94	0.91	1.09
		F	**0.96**	1.15	0.96	1.08	1.07	0.88	0.90	0.91
151	Malignant neoplasm of stomach	M	**1.12**	1.11	1.13	1.08	1.17	1.07	1.03	1.00
		F	**1.07**	1.07	1.15	1.12	1.20	0.88	0.97	1.10
152	Malignant neoplasm of small intestine, including duodenum	M	**1.40**	0.57	1.80	1.00	1.25	2.00	1.50	0.73
		F	**1.37**	1.00	1.43	3.00	1.20	1.00	2.00	1.25
153	Malignant neoplasm of colon	M	**1.32**	1.46	1.43	1.52	1.39	1.16	1.15	1.15
		F	**1.36**	1.45	1.47	1.48	1.57	1.21	1.24	1.34
154	Malignant neoplasm of rectum, rectosigmoid junction and anus	M	**1.64**	1.44	1.86	1.68	1.79	1.47	1.49	1.59
		F	**1.57**	1.48	1.69	1.48	1.76	1.63	1.47	1.40
155	Malignant neoplasm of liver and intrahepatic bile-ducts	M	**0.81**	0.75	1.03	0.76	0.57	0.84	0.77	0.86
		F	**0.76**	0.79	0.69	0.71	0.39	0.86	0.85	0.69
156	Malignant neoplasm of gallbladder and extrahepatic bile ducts	M	**1.41**	1.37	0.97	1.61	2.31	1.56	0.74	2.06
		F	**1.26**	1.37	1.25	1.55	2.50	1.03	0.94	1.13
157	Malignant neoplasm of pancreas	M	**0.94**	0.81	0.85	1.03	1.14	0.87	0.92	0.89
		F	**0.92**	0.92	0.89	0.92	0.98	0.87	0.85	0.95
158	Malignant neoplasm of retroperitoneum and peritoneum	M	**1.09**	0.90	0.67	1.33	8.00	1.40	0.82	0.44
		F	**1.39**	0.25	1.33	3.60	1.50	1.00	1.14	3.00
159	Malignant neoplasm of other and ill-defined sites within the digestive organs and peritoneum	M	**0.44**	0.73	0.12	0.52	0.19	0.48	0.66	0.54
		F	**0.51**	0.57	0.36	0.46	0.41	0.46	0.65	0.54
160	Malignant neoplasm of nasal cavities, middle ear and accessory sinuses	M	**1.88**	0.90	1.08	4.75	2.29	1.78	1.71	3.17
		F	**1.90**	6.00	0.60	1.33	5.00	2.00	1.62	2.17

* See explanatory note on page 3 regarding apparent decrease of North East Thames figures.

England and Wales regional health authorities

South West Thames	Wessex	Oxford	South Western	West Midlands	Mersey	North Western	Wales		Site description	ICD (9th Revision) number
1.35	**1.54**	**1.55**	**1.40**	**1.51**	**1.51**	**1.50**	**1.41**	M	All malignant neoplasms	140-208
1.47	**1.67**	**1.66**	**1.56**	**1.61**	**1.63**	**1.63**	**1.59**	F		
6.00	4.00	19.00	12.00	3.50	1.00	1.67	7.00	M	Malignant neoplasm of lip	140
:	:	2.50	:	1.50	1.00	:	4.00	F		
1.89	1.33	1.25	1.18	2.10	1.57	1.90	2.25	M	Malignant neoplasm of tongue	141
1.00	0.83	2.33	1.37	1.43	2.43	0.53	1.57	F		
1.80	1.37	0.50	1.00	0.93	3.00	1.40	1.86	M	Malignant neoplasm of major	142
3.50	1.50	3.00	1.00	6.33	1.71	1.80	7.67	F	salivary glands	
1.50	0.67	3.00	2.50	0.80	2.00	1.43	1.33	M	Malignant neoplasm of gum	143
1.00	0.80	0.67	-	2.00	-	3.00	1.00	F		
1.00	4.00	1.33	1.40	1.55	1.64	5.60	13.00	M	Malignant neoplasm of floor of	144
1.00	1.50	:	0.75	3.00	1.67	1.50	1.33	F	mouth	
0.80	7.00	6.00	1.33	4.17	1.78	1.78	1.00	M	Malignant neoplasm of other and	145
2.40	2.75	6.00	1.00	8.33	0.75	1.33	2.00	F	unspecified parts of mouth	
1.00	0.67	2.00	1.18	1.71	3.17	1.95	1.27	M	Malignant neoplasm of oropharynx	146
2.50	1.50	1.67	3.00	1.83	3.00	1.44	1.67	F		
1.60	1.00	2.00	0.14	1.31	0.67	1.00	2.33	M	Malignant neoplasm of	147
0.75	:	0.80	0.50	1.20	0.20	1.40	0.80	F	nasopharynx	
3.00	1.00	0.71	0.70	2.25	2.56	2.67	1.00	M	Malignant neoplasm of	148
2.50	0.75	0.60	1.67	2.00	0.56	1.00	1.00	F	hypopharynx	
2.00	1.00	0.80	0.62	0.37	0.86	1.43	1.67	M	Malignant neoplasm of other and	149
1.00	:	1.00	1.00	0.37	1.00	0.62	3.00	F	ill-defined sites within the lip oral cavity and pharynx	
0.99	1.25	0.56	0.91	0.92	0.92	0.98	1.20	M	Malignant neoplasm of oesophagus	150
0.85	1.05	0.95	0.88	0.93	1.01	0.98	0.80	F		
1.02	1.20	1.25	1.00	1.28	1.31	1.21	0.95	M	Malignant neoplasm of stomach	151
0.85	1.11	1.29	0.96	1.10	1.19	1.12	1.01	F		
2.00	1.57	1.43	0.75	2.27	1.86	1.00	1.37	M	Malignant neoplasm of small	152
1.29	0.83	1.25	0.64	1.50	0.62	1.75	3.00	F	intestine, including duodenum	
1.20	1.62	1.36	1.31	1.39	1.47	1.28	0.98	M	Malignant neoplasm of colon	153
1.25	1.41	1.45	1.22	1.38	1.32	1.51	1.16	F		
1.41	1.74	1.59	1.55	1.78	1.65	1.47	1.94	M	Malignant neoplasm of rectum,	154
1.35	1.81	1.74	1.67	1.34	1.68	1.68	1.83	F	rectosigmoid junction and anus	
0.62	0.93	0.67	0.82	0.65	0.90	0.92	0.98	M	Malignant neoplasm of liver and	155
0.77	1.14	0.48	1.16	0.67	0.72	0.80	0.79	F	intrahepatic bile-ducts	
1.33	0.83	1.27	1.67	1.44	1.33	1.67	1.42	M	Malignant neoplasm of gallbladder	156
0.92	1.11	1.60	1.12	1.16	1.21	1.41	1.45	F	and extrahepatic bile ducts	
0.97	0.95	0.94	0.83	0.97	1.03	1.06	0.91	M	Malignant neoplasm of pancreas	157
0.81	1.02	0.93	0.99	0.94	0.97	1.04	0.72	F		
1.33	1.14	1.00	0.37	1.00	1.75	1.10	9.00	M	Malignant neoplasm of	158
1.00	1.67	1.00	0.58	0.70	1.83	1.83	6.00	F	retroperitoneum and peritoneum	
0.41	1.05	0.08	0.24	-	0.07	0.61	0.90	M	Malignant neoplasm of other and	159
0.72	0.72	0.22	0.58	-	0.06	0.62	1.10	F	ill-defined sites within the digestive organs and peritoneum	
1.00	1.17	1.71	2.67	1.31	12.00	2.87	2.50	M	Malignant neoplasm of nasal	160
2.50	4.33	0.67	1.50	2.25	1.33	1.00	2.67	F	cavities, middle ear and accessory sinuses	

Appendix C Series MB1 no. 19

Appendix C Incidence to mortality ratios - *continued*

ICD (9th Revision) number	Site description		England and Wales	Northern	Yorkshire	Trent	East Anglian	North West Thames	North East Thames*	South East Thames
161	Malignant neoplasm of larynx	M F	**2.21** **1.91**	1.83 2.33	2.06 2.70	2.23 2.43	2.94 *2.40*	2.56 *0.70*	1.74 *1.36*	1.79 *1.42*
162	Malignant neoplasm of trachea, bronchus and lung	M F	**0.97** **1.00**	0.99 0.97	0.97 1.00	1.04 1.08	0.98 1.16	0.87 0.81	0.85 0.90	0.86 0.92
163	Malignant neoplasm of pleura	M F	**1.40** **1.52**	0.98 *1.60*	1.37 *1.00*	0.70 *1.14*	*1.64* *2.00*	2.25 *1.00*	1.62 *1.25*	1.30 *2.33*
164	Malignant neoplasm of thymus heart and mediastinum	M F	**1.86** **1.46**	7.00 :	*0.57* *1.00*	5.00 :	*0.25* *0.67*	2.50 *1.50*	*0.80* *1.67*	4.00 *4.50*
165	Malignant neoplasm of other and ill-defined sites within the respiratory system and intrathoracic organs	M F	**0.87** **0.33**	- -	- -	- -	: -	- -	- -	- -
170	Malignant neoplasm of bone and articular cartilage	M F	**1.75** **2.06**	*1.86* *2.20*	*1.44* *1.50*	1.92 1.93	*2.75* *1.50*	2.12 *1.22*	*1.36* *3.40*	2.09 *2.80*
171	Malignant neoplasm of connective and other soft tissue	M F	**1.59** **1.60**	2.11 2.21	1.14 1.41	1.41 1.45	2.18 1.60	1.62 1.33	1.25 1.40	1.08 1.37
172	Malignant melanoma of skin	M F	**2.23** **3.07**	3.41 2.48	2.14 4.06	2.13 2.92	2.20 3.72	2.20 1.98	2.09 1.84	1.49 2.57
173	Other malignant neoplasm of skin	M F	**61.81** **69.32**	39.05 50.07	82.43 136.37	71.22 91.23	70.64 209.00	59.50 34.07	40.06 37.80	53.21 37.29
174	Malignant neoplasm of female breast	F	**1.67**	1.67	1.61	1.71	1.72	1.59	1.51	1.40
175	Malignant neoplasm of male breast	M	**1.50**	*0.60*	*0.89*	2.67	*1.44*	*1.13*	*1.00*	*0.83*
179	Malignant neoplasm of uterus, part unspecified	F	**0.72**	0.68	1.20	1.51	0.21	-	-	-
180	Malignant neoplasm of cervix uteri	F	**2.02**	1.93	2.25	1.98	1.96	1.46	1.61	1.59
181	Malignant neoplasm of placenta	F	**2.20**	:	1.00	:	-	:	:	-
182	Malignant neoplasm of body of uterus	F	**3.71**	3.73	4.62	4.13	3.76	3.23	3.39	3.91
183	Malignant neoplasm of ovary and other uterine adnexa	F	**1.17**	1.31	1.29	1.22	1.45	1.08	1.02	1.05
184	Malignant neoplasm of other and unspecified female genital organs	F	**1.88**	2.24	1.83	2.22	1.86	1.34	1.47	1.38
185	Malignant neoplasm of prostate	M	**1.48**	1.58	1.56	1.56	1.56	1.31	1.25	1.26
186	Malignant neoplasm of testis	M	**8.18**	7.44	5.30	7.31	9.60	8.86	8.57	6.50
187	Malignant neoplasm of penis and other male genital organs	M	**2.68**	2.12	4.33	1.86	*6.00*	*1.75*	2.50	*1.50*
188	Malignant neoplasm of bladder	M F	**2.14** **1.86**	2.07 1.76	1.99 1.97	2.24 2.23	2.50 1.89	2.30 1.94	1.88 1.42	1.70 1.39
189	Malignant neoplasm of kidney and other and unspecified urinary organs	M F	**1.38** **1.41**	1.36 1.33	1.46 1.55	1.29 1.46	1.59 1.39	1.09 1.70	1.58 1.17	1.35 1.34
190	Malignant neoplasm of eye	M F	**1.92** **2.12**	*1.62* 2.67	*1.62* *1.33*	2.33 2.67	: 4.50	3.14 3.25	5.00 *1.33*	*1.86* 2.67
191	Malignant neoplasm of brain	M F	**1.12** **1.05**	1.12 0.93	1.10 1.18	1.19 1.10	1.29 1.38	1.03 1.10	0.84 0.85	1.04 0.96

* See explanatory note on page 3 regarding apparent decrease of North East Thames figures.

Series MB1 no. 19 Appendix C

South West Thames	Wessex	Oxford	South Western	West Midlands	Mersey	North Western	Wales		Site description	ICD (9th Revision) number
1.97	3.04	2.57	1.61	2.49	1.97	2.41	3.03	M	Malignant neoplasm of larynx	161
1.54	1.75	1.67	1.60	3.56	1.14	2.18	3.22	F		
0.92	1.04	1.00	0.86	1.04	1.06	1.05	0.96	M	Malignant neoplasm of trachea,	162
0.90	1.07	1.07	0.88	1.03	1.14	1.12	1.06	F	bronchus and lung	
1.10	1.60	1.00	1.30	1.78	2.00	2.67	0.94	M	Malignant neoplasm of pleura	163
0.75	0.75	1.67	2.50	1.50	3.33	2.20	4.00	F		
8.00	2.00	:	1.50	0.89	:	:	2.00	M	Malignant neoplasm of thymus	164
3.00	1.33	1.00	1.00	0.67	:	1.00	1.00	F	heart and mediastinum	
-	0.50	-	-	-	-	2.00	1.50	M	Malignant neoplasm of other and	165
-	-	-	-	-	-	-	:	F	ill-defined sites within the respiratory system and intrathoracic organs	
1.40	2.00	8.00	1.86	0.95	0.43	2.00	2.67	M	Malignant neoplasm of bone and	170
4.00	1.75	2.20	0.75	1.27	3.33	1.44	4.50	F	articular cartilage	
1.30	4.11	0.72	1.50	1.89	1.70	2.17	1.47	M	Malignant neoplasm of connective	171
1.28	1.39	1.00	1.29	1.83	2.00	2.85	2.30	F	and other soft tissue	
2.03	3.24	1.57	2.04	2.79	1.50	3.17	2.50	M	Malignant melanoma of skin	172
3.02	4.90	3.45	3.65	3.61	2.64	2.83	3.15	F		
53.12	50.40	74.91	84.25	78.14	81.10	80.20	38.90	M	Other malignant neoplasm of skin	173
121.00	57.36	59.18	58.20	78.11	91.00	91.46	85.62	F		
1.62	1.94	1.71	1.78	1.75	1.75	1.71	1.76	F	Malignant neoplasm of female breast	174
8.00	2.00	4.00	1.12	0.64	1.67	10.00	3.33	M	Malignant neoplasm of male breast	175
-	1.44	-	0.84	0.74	0.62	2.03	1.47	F	Malignant neoplasm of uterus, part unspecified	179
2.16	2.49	1.97	2.55	2.74	1.88	1.80	2.15	F	Malignant neoplasm of cervix uteri	180
-	-	:	:	1.00	-	:	-	F	Malignant neoplasm of placenta	181
5.72	3.17	4.37	2.69	3.61	4.15	3.39	3.43	F	Malignant neoplasm of body of uterus	182
1.12	1.27	1.45	0.90	1.20	1.21	1.20	1.22	F	Malignant neoplasm of ovary and other uterine adnexa	183
1.46	1.92	2.28	1.70	1.82	2.22	2.28	2.43	F	Malignant neoplasm of other and unspecified female genital organs	184
1.38	1.66	1.67	1.37	1.65	1.55	1.52	1.42	M	Malignant neoplasm of prostate	185
11.67	15.00	14.00	9.78	15.00	2.85	7.09	7.00	M	Malignant neoplasm of testis	186
5.00	2.71	2.43	2.22	2.71	7.00	1.86	6.25	M	Malignant neoplasm of penis and other male genital organs	187
1.85	2.41	2.65	1.87	2.18	2.25	2.40	2.57	M	Malignant neoplasm of bladder	188
1.46	1.86	2.36	1.82	1.81	2.60	2.03	2.33	F		
1.28	1.49	1.56	1.22	1.37	1.76	1.53	1.24	M	Malignant neoplasm of kidney and	189
1.21	1.41	2.04	1.35	1.24	1.12	1.53	1.81	F	other and unspecified urinary organs	
3.80	1.57	1.00	1.37	0.75	1.33	1.42	2.40	M	Malignant neoplasm of eye	190
2.00	2.00	1.00	5.00	3.00	1.00	1.55	2.50	F		
1.04	1.19	1.15	0.86	1.21	1.33	1.32	1.14	M	Malignant neoplasm of brain	191
1.01	1.00	0.95	0.80	1.00	1.12	1.21	1.60	F		

Appendix C Incidence to mortality ratios - *continued*

ICD (9th Revision) number	Site description		England and Wales	Northern	Yorkshire	Trent	East Anglian	North West Thames	North East Thames*	South East Thames
				\multicolumn{8}{c}{Regional health authority of residence}
192	Malignant neoplasm of other and unspecified parts of nervous system	M F	**1.70** **1.96**	*4.00* *4.50*	*3.00* -	*3.00* *0.75*	*1.00* *0.33*	*1.00* *5.00*	*1.00* *0.50*	*7.00* :
193	Malignant neoplasm of thyroid gland	M F	**2.27** **2.39**	*2.20* *2.53*	*1.80* *2.92*	*1.79* *3.69*	: *4.29*	*3.00* *1.96*	*4.00* *1.80*	*1.43* *1.41*
194	Malignant neoplasm of other endocrine glands and related structures	M F	**1.16** **1.48**	*0.60* *1.00*	*0.57* *0.75*	*2.00* *4.00*	*0.40* *4.00*	*4.00* *1.00*	*1.33* *1.75*	*2.33* *1.33*
195	Malignant neoplasm of other and ill-defined sites	M F	**0.90** **0.98**	*1.89* *2.29*	*0.42* *0.82*	*2.21* *1.64*	*0.33* *1.00*	*0.14* *0.47*	*0.27* *0.12*	*0.44* *0.12*
196	Secondary and unspecified malignant neoplasm of lymph nodes	M F	: :	: :	: :	: :	: :	: :	: :	: :
197	Secondary malignant neoplasm of respiratory and digestive systems	M F	: :	: :	: :	: :	: :	: :	: :	: :
198	Secondary malignant neoplasm of other specified sites	M F	: :	: :	: :	: :	: :	: :	: :	: :
199	Malignant neoplasm without specification of site	M F	**0.50** **0.49**	0.52 0.60	0.49 0.51	0.52 0.57	0.39 0.36	0.41 0.32	0.44 0.48	0.37 0.31
200	Lymphosarcoma and reticulosarcoma	M F	**2.18** **1.83**	*1.55* *1.80*	*5.43* *6.67*	*3.11* *2.10*	*0.43* *0.75*	*1.80* *1.60*	*1.29* *1.17*	*1.21* *1.10*
201	Hodgkin's disease	M F	**2.49** **2.60**	1.59 2.73	1.96 4.86	2.63 1.86	2.60 7.00	2.62 2.45	2.80 2.15	2.57 1.82
202	Other malignant neoplasm of lymphoid and histiocytic tissue	M F	**1.50** **1.51**	1.55 1.95	1.04 1.41	1.72 1.34	2.08 1.62	1.47 1.75	1.21 1.12	1.32 1.59
203	Multiple myeloma and immunoproliferative neoplasms	M F	**1.14** **1.07**	1.05 1.49	1.05 0.88	1.48 1.25	1.25 0.98	1.16 0.96	0.89 0.95	0.94 1.01
204-208	All leukaemias	M F	**1.13** **1.11**	1.30 1.11	1.02 1.14	1.34 1.53	1.31 1.29	1.18 0.99	1.04 0.95	1.01 0.95
204	Lymphoid leukaemia	M F	**1.35** **1.34**	1.47 1.43	1.07 1.44	1.52 1.82	1.32 1.60	1.86 1.36	1.55 1.21	1.25 1.04
205	Myeloid leukaemia	M F	**0.97** **0.97**	1.08 0.93	0.94 1.00	1.16 1.41	1.26 1.21	0.75 0.80	0.74 0.71	0.81 0.89
206	Monocytic leukaemia	M F	**0.87** **1.31**	: *1.67*	*0.75* *1.33*	*2.33* *3.00*	: *1.50*	*0.50* -	*0.33* :	*0.33* *1.33*
207	Other specified leukaemia	M F	0.63 *0.86*	*1.50* *1.50*	*0.50* :	*1.25* *1.00*	*1.00* -	- *0.33*	*0.33* *0.50*	*0.50* *1.00*
208	Leukaemia of unspecified cell type	M F	**1.47** **1.08**	*2.00* *1.25*	*1.56* *1.18*	*1.80* *0.50*	*1.00* *0.67*	*2.12* *1.37*	*2.57* *1.78*	*1.80* *0.91*

* See explanatory note on page 3 regarding apparent decrease of North East Thames figures.

Series MB1 no. 19 Appendix C

South West Thames	Wessex	Oxford	South Western	West Midlands	Mersey	North Western	Wales		Site description	ICD (9th Revision) number
:	1.00	0.50	1.00	0.80	2.00	2.00	2.00	M	Malignant neoplasm of other and unspecified parts of nervous system	192
4.00	2.00	2.00	:	1.00	3.00	:	1.67	F		
2.25	2.00	3.00	1.92	2.09	1.37	3.60	3.00	M	Malignant neoplasm of thyroid gland	193
5.80	2.09	3.11	1.68	2.04	3.40	1.90	3.00	F		
2.50	0.75	0.57	2.00	0.40	1.00	1.50	:	M	Malignant neoplasm of other endocrine glands and related structures	194
3.00	6.00	1.20	2.50	0.67	1.33	0.50	4.00	F		
0.58	1.78	0.12	0.93	-	0.86	1.10	3.86	M	Malignant neoplasm of other and ill-defined sites	195
0.75	2.53	0.09	1.37	-	0.54	1.22	2.47	F		
:	:	:	:	:	:	:	:	M	Secondary and unspecified malignant neoplasm of lymph nodes	196
:	:	:	:	:	:	:	:	F		
:	:	:	:	:	:	:	:	M	Secondary malignant neoplasm of respiratory and digestive systems	197
:	:	:	:	:	:	:	:	F		
:	:	:	:	:	:	:	:	M	Secondary malignant neoplasm of other specified sites	198
:	:	:	:	:	:	:	:	F		
0.32	0.50	0.30	0.71	0.94	0.43	0.36	0.51	M	Malignant neoplasm without specification of site	199
0.35	0.61	0.29	0.67	0.90	0.44	0.33	0.41	F		
0.93	1.45	5.33	3.35	1.93	2.60	2.55	3.00	M	Lymphosarcoma and reticulosarcoma	200
0.37	1.11	1.71	8.40	1.87	3.25	2.89	0.67	F		
2.22	2.41	3.00	2.83	2.70	2.13	3.27	2.58	M	Hodgkin's disease	201
2.12	2.00	2.00	2.12	2.05	4.00	5.00	3.10	F		
1.68	1.64	1.34	1.84	1.48	1.21	1.91	1.24	M	Other malignant neoplasm of lymphoid and histiocytic tissue	202
1.74	1.54	1.06	1.74	1.41	1.75	1.82	1.28	F		
0.94	0.99	1.21	1.67	1.22	0.75	1.21	1.29	M	Multiple myeloma and immunoproliferative neoplasms	203
1.03	1.27	0.76	1.14	0.92	0.89	1.22	1.42	F		
0.80	1.22	0.95	1.69	0.51	1.04	1.45	1.33	M	All leukaemias	204-208
0.88	1.37	1.04	1.53	0.57	0.92	1.33	1.26	F		
1.06	1.60	1.17	2.55	0.71	0.86	1.27	1.46	M	Lymphoid leukaemia	204
1.04	1.93	1.30	2.09	0.70	0.89	1.37	1.58	F		
0.62	1.08	0.86	1.41	0.36	1.07	1.71	1.22	M	Myeloid leukaemia	205
0.75	1.15	0.90	1.20	0.55	0.82	1.48	0.99	F		
0.33	0.75	1.00	0.67	0.37	2.00	3.00	0.67	M	Monocytic leukaemia	206
0.50	0.75	1.00	1.43	0.60	:	1.00	:	F		
0.80	0.33	-	0.50	-	-	0.50	1.00	M	Other specified leukaemia	207
-	2.00	-	:	0.67	1.00	0.25	:	F		
0.85	0.60	0.75	1.17	0.55	5.00	1.75	2.00	M	Leukaemia of unspecified cell type	208
1.00	1.17	1.40	1.25	0.15	1.67	0.62	8.00	F		